PSYCHIATRIC DISORDERS
IN OBSTETRICS

Psychiatric Disorders in Obstetrics

A. A. BAKER
M.D. D.P.M.

Consultant Psychiatrist and
Medical Administrator, Banstead Hospital

Consultant Psychiatrist to
St Mary Abbots Hospital

Consultant in charge of the
Mother and Baby Unit, Downview Hospital

BLACKWELL SCIENTIFIC PUBLICATIONS
OXFORD AND EDINBURGH

Set by
SANTYPE LTD, SALISBURY
Printed in Great Britain by
THE SALISBURY PRESS LTD, SALISBURY
and bound by
THE KEMP HALL BINDERY, OXFORD

Contents

Foreword

I feel proud to have been asked to contribute a preface to this book since I have played a part in persuading Dr Baker to write it. I was so impressed by a lecture given by Dr Baker some years ago at the Royal Society of Medicine on the psychiatric problems of pregnancy and the puerperium that I said to him afterwards it was really his duty to make the fruits of his experience available to a wider audience. I am sure that all the readers of this book will agree with me that it is a most valuable and practical contribution to this important yet strangely neglected subject.

Dr Baker's special interest in these problems dates back, he tells me, to 1951, and his personal experience must be unique in this country. The internationally well known Mother and Baby Unit was opened at Banstead, on Dr Baker's initiative, in 1958, after three years of research on the social problems of young mothers after they had left psychiatric hospital. Taking one syndrome alone, between two and three hundred mothers suffering from schizophrenia have since passed through the Banstead Mother and Baby Unit; and in addition, there have of course been many other mothers suffering from depression or toxic confusional states. Mothers suffering from a neurosis— and many such sufferers have passed through Dr Baker's hands —have, with relatively few exceptions, been treated on an outpatient basis.

I know of no other psychiatrist in Great Britain who has had such a wealth of personal clinical experience concerning the psychiatric problems of pregnancy and the puerperium. Although this book has been written primarily for the benefit of general practitioners, obstetricians and psychiatrists I can also commend it to medical students and midwives. As readers will find, Dr Baker has at his command, in addition to his vast experience, a clear and easy style that is refreshingly free from jargon.

I am sure that all who read this book will join me in congratulating Dr Baker on an outstandingly perceptive and balanced monograph. We may not all agree with all he says; but we can all agree that his opinions and advice must be treated with deep respect.

28 December 1966   Prof. Desmond Curran
                                    C.B.E M.B. B.Ch.
                                    F.R.C.P. D.P.M.

CHAPTER ONE

Introduction

Quot homines tot sententiae

Birth is the most important event in the life of the individual and the family. No other event has such obvious physical, emotional and social repercussions on the woman or her immediate associates. It is not surprising that such an event should be surrounded with a multitude of myths, old wives tales and prejudices. With the advent of a more scientific attitude in medicine one would have expected that much more precise information would now be available and that many previous misconceptions would have been removed. In practice, this is not the case. It is possible to find even in the recent literature completely differing opinions on almost all psychiatric aspects of the problem. For example, there are still some who consider that there is a specific entity, puerperal psychosis, and indeed this is recognized in the International Nomenclature. On the other hand, it is probable that the majority of psychiatrists now consider there is no such entity, but that the usual psychiatric illnesses are merely precipitated and modified by this particular situation and stress. There are equally great divergencies of opinion between those who consider the illnesses are largely due to physical causes, including hormonal changes; and those who consider that the essence of the disturbance lies in the patient's emotional life. In 1964 one author advised that mother and baby should always be separated, while many writers were advising that they should be kept together if at all possible. Lastly, in the field of prognosis, we can find those who believe that the prognosis in the puerperium is worse for a given illness, and others who consider the prognosis is better in this situation. We must consider some of the facts and then attempt to understand the reasons for these differing opinions.

It is reasonably certain that there have been considerable

changes in the forms of mental illness in the puerperium in the last thirty years. Before the advent of effective antibiotics toxic-confusional psychoses, secondary to major infection, were relatively common in the puerperium. For example, in 1931 Solomons wrote that toxaemia and sepsis were the commonest factors in puerperal psychoses, and Piker in 1938 assessed the aetiology in a series of 981 cases, and found that 35 per cent of these were due to toxic exhaustion. A very similar incidence was found by Cruickshank two years later. Even as late as 1943, Jacobs reported 50 per cent of physical factors in his series. It is striking that in 1955 Tetlow was able to report no difference between a group of patients with puerperal psychoses and those mothers without psychiatric illness in the puerperium, the incidence of infection in both groups being 7 per cent. Equally striking were Hemphill's findings. He compared a series between the years 1938 and 1948, when the incidence of physical factors was 20 per cent, and another group between 1948 and 1952 when no such conditions were found. Thus it seems likely that the total number of psychoses in the puerperium has been reduced over the years in those countries where antibiotics are freely available, owing to the control of toxic conditions. This possibility would be confirmed by the figures given by Herzen of 2·5 psychoses per thousand births in 1906 compared with Tetlow's figures of 1·5 per thousand in 1955.

On first considerations, it is difficult to understand the differing opinions on the prognosis for puerperal psychoses. The most striking example lies in the case of schizophrenia. Hemphill, for example, considers the illness has a singularly bad prognosis in the puerperium, while Martin found that all her cases responded well to treatment. Equally opposed are the views of those who find major precipitants of the illness in the personality of the patient, compared with those who have failed to find any such differences. Zilboorg for example is identified with the opinion that pre-existing personality conflicts and attitudes underlie puerperal mental illness, but neither Anderson in 1933 nor Martin in 1958 found evidence in the pre-psychotic personality of their patients to explain the subsequent breakdown. From the clinical point of view it is extremely difficult to believe that the previous personality can play a major part in the development of the psychoses, though there is no doubt it plays a part in neurotic illness. It is a common clinical observation that a woman may have a psychosis after some of her children but no such psychosis after others, when all other stresses seem to be unchanged. It is difficult in this situation to believe that the previous personality is significant other than in determining the type of symptom evidenced.

Similarly conflicting opinions can be found concerning the role of the endocrine system. For example, the French workers, Delay, Corteel and Boittelle, describe a series of cases in which hormonal functions were studied by means of endometrial biopsies. They found that the one assessment is of little value unless the patients previous hormonal levels, both during her normal cycle and in the puerperium, are known.

It is worth while giving further consideration to some of the reasons for the varying opinions found, as this will no doubt help us to a better understanding of the illnesses and also lead to a better assessment of the literature. Firstly we must briefly consider the historical background. It is perhaps unfortunate that the first case is that described by Hippocrates. He noted the case of a patient who developed a psychosis after the birth of twins. This patient became delirious and eventually died. He attempted to find the cause of illnesses such as this in abnormalities in the discharges following childbirth or abnormalities in the breast during lactation. It is understandable that the occurrence of severe uterine infections following childbirth, or breast abscesses, both of which could lead to severe toxaemia and delirium, would tend to strengthen such a hypothesis. It is more likely, however, that the Bible has had a much more profound effect, particularly on the ordinary woman, than any remarks by Hippocrates. For example in Genesis we find '. . . in sorrow thou shalt bring forth children . . .' and these words must have echoed in the ears of many girls from their earliest years, and would have had added significance for those generations in the Victorian era when church attendance and the acceptance of dogma were the current social pattern. A more scientific study of the problem was made by Marcé in the middle of the nineteenth century. He was one of the first to note the emotional changes in pregnancy, during which some stable women develop anxiety for the first time, while previously anxious women may become calm and confident. He separated his patients into those suffering from the immediate puerperal illnesses, in which the onset developed within six weeks, and the later group which he associated with lactation. It is of interest that Marcé has been quoted to support two quite contrary opinions. There are those who note his comment that all the symptons of post partum mental illness can be found in other mental illnesses, while others, for example, Hamilton, consider that the chief emphasis in Marcé's work was to the effect that the syndromes were different in puerperal cases.

Another factor underlying the varying opinions on puerperal mental illness is the variations in the clinical picture produced by the puerperium. In the first week or two of the puerperium considerable emotional lability is common. In the first week considerable changes in hormone level occur and the woman is also adjusting to the presence of the new member of her family. All these factors tend to produce marked swings in the clinical picture. Tears may be present one day, laughter the next. Frank psychosis may be reported in the morning, normality by evening. It is clear that in this situation dramatic 'cures' are possible. These may merely represent the return to normality occurring as the patient's natural resources reassert themselves. In pregnancy too, the changes of mood which go with the condition will modify the clinical picture in many cases. Certainly, anyone who tries to predict the course of pregnancy and the puerperium from examination made in the first few months is likely to be wrong. Similarly those who make predictions in the middle three months—the months of emotional stability—may be surprised at the results of their follow-up. The obstetrician and the psychiatrist, both of whom may see the patient for a limited period during the total cycle, may have a very biased view of the patient's stability and resources. The general practitioner, however, particularly if he knows the patient from her earlier years and perhaps the family history too, may be in a better position to observe changes and assess their significance by making comparisons with his patient's normal way of life.

A further perusal of the literature suggests that very conflicting opinions can be obtained as a result of the selection of different groups of patients. There are undoubted differences in the personalities, cultural background, type of illness and also the prognosis in those patients who will attend a private psychiatrist, those who go to the teaching hospital, those who attend the out-patient clinic or those who have to be admitted under order to a mental hospital. Moreover, since treatment facilities, public opinion, and many other factors have changed dramatically within the last few years, it is not possible to compare the results of treatment even between those treated one year previously and those treated in the current year. As others have noted, this particular group of psychiatric patients have often had their initial examination made by someone with limited psychiatric experience, frequently the obstetric houseman. Much will depend on his attitude towards mental illness whether the patient is referred promptly for further care or whether, as one writer described his practice 'the patient should be observed to see if the delusions will go away'. As will be noted repeatedly throughout this book, the assessment of the patient, her treatment, and the ultimate prognosis for herself, her child and her family, all depend on the willingness of those caring for her to make a full assessment of her condition and all the factors which play a part.

REFERENCES

ANDERSON E.W. (1933) A study of the sexual life in psychoses associated with childbirth. *J. Ment. Sci.* **79**, 137.

CRUICKSHANK W.H. (1940) Psychoses associated with pregnancy and the puerperium. *Canad. Med. Ass. J.* **43**, 571.
DELAY J., CORTEEL A. & LAINÉ B. (1953) Traitement des psychoses du post partum. *Ann. Endocr.* **14**, 428.
GENESIS, chapter III, verse 16.
HEMPHILL R.E. (1952) Incidence and nature of puerperal psychiatric illness. *Brit. Med. J.* **2**, 1232.
HERZER G. (1906) *Allg. Z. Psychiat.* **63**, 244.
JACOBS B. (1943) Aetiological factors and reaction types in psychoses following childbirth. *J. Ment. Sci.* **89**, 242.
MARCÉ L.V. (1858) Traité de la folie des femmes enceintes. Paris.
MARTIN M.E. (1958) Puerperal mental illness: a follow-up study of 75 cases. *Brit. Med. J.* **2**, 773.
PIKER P. (1938) Psychoses complicating childbearing. *Amer. J. Obstet. Gynec.* **35**, 901.
SOLOMONS B. (1931) *J. Ment. Sci.* **77**, 701.
TETLOW C. (1955) Psychoses of childbearing. *J. Ment. Sci.* **101**, 629.
ZILBOORG G. (1928) *Amer. J. Obstet. Gynec.* **15**, 145.

The following books are suggested as further reading:

FOULKES S.H. & ANTHONY E.J. (1965) *Group Psychotherapy*. [Gives further information on this subject]
HAMILTON J.A. (1962) *Post Partum Psychiatric Problems*. St. Louis. [Reveals some current American attitudes]
JANSSON, BENGT (1964) *Psychic Insufficiencies associated with Childbirth*. [Gives a considerable amount of information about the situation in Denmark]
MAYER-GROSS W., SLATER E. & ROTH M. (1960) *Clinical Psychiatry*. [For further clinical information, particularly concerning organic factors and genetics]
SARGANT W. & SLATER E. (1963) *Introduction to Physical Methods of Treatment in Psychiatry*. [For further guidance on physical treatment]

CHAPTER TWO

The Human Framework

Before we consider the patient herself and her problems during pregnancy, childbirth and the puerperium we should give further thought to those who set the stage for her at these vital periods in her life. The people primarily concerned are, of course, her husband, her mother and other relatives, the general practitioner, the midwife and the obstetrician. We will consider each of these in turn. Each has their own personality and attitudes, their own anxieties, hopes and previous experience to bring to the situation. Psychiatry is always concerned with the relationships between people and emotional relationships are always tested when strong feelings are aroused. The strongest possible feelings are aroused by childbearing, intense love and intense fear can both be present. The woman giving birth will always take the centre of the stage and experience the deepest emotions. Her ability to play her part successfully will depend on the understanding shown by those playing a supporting role.

The husband

It is too easy to see the wife as the centre of the stage and overlook her husband's role and her husband's anxieties. Awareness of the part he plays is now much more common, however, though it is only recently that he has been able to be present during labour in maternity units, and few are designed to make this a routine. Nevertheless, it is essential that his personality and reactions should be known to the obstetrician or midwife and equally important that the information he can give about his wife should be available to those who will care for her.

Her own account of her previous personality, previous illnesses and reaction to the present pregnancy can all be coloured by the current emotional state to such an extent that a completely erroneous impression is received. The husband is usually the person who can most easily place the history given by his wife in its proper perspective. Other relatives can be helpful but the patient's own mother will often give a history biased by her own emotional attitudes. The majority of husbands will support their wives, relieve their anxieties and co-operate to the full with all treatment. Nevertheless, their faith in those caring for their wives may be severely disturbed not only by unexpected physical complications but also by unexpected psychiatric symptoms. If, for example, the patient's symptoms are paranoid in nature, the husband may automatically accept his wife's account of her 'ill treatment' and her medical advisers will find it very difficult to maintain a satisfactory relationship with either. When things go wrong it is inevitable that the husband will either tend to blame himself, his wife, or those caring for her and, in general, the more faithful and loving the husband, the more likely he is, unless he is given adequate explanation of the situation, to blame those caring for his wife. Most men experience very considerable anxiety when their wives have children and should she develop psychiatric symptoms his stress will be considerably increased by this new, unknown, and often frightening factor. It is common to find that women with psychiatric symptoms have husbands who also show obvious evidence of anxiety and it may then be tempting to believe that the wife's condition is due to her anxious husband or even to assume that his inadequacy underlies her difficulties.

A short discussion with the husband will usually give some idea of his personality and also his attitudes towards his wife. He will usually reveal his anxieties and the way in which he reveals them will show whether he is essentially self-centred or primarily concerned in helping his wife. It may be obvious to the casual observer that there are some stresses in the marriage or some unusual circumstances. Marked age disparity whether the husband is younger or older will usually be found to be an expression of some emotional problem in either or both partners. Some 'managing' women marry men who are willing to be managed. A woman becomes relatively helpless and dependent on others at childbirth and for a time afterwards, and this type of 'managing' woman may then have considerable difficulties and, her husband, who until this time has relied upon her, may find it difficult to assert himself. Many husbands have little idea of the role they should play when their wife has a child. A frank discussion of sex relations during pregnancy and in the puerperium, of the management of sickness or food fads, and the need to support his wife and give emotional warmth to other children, will help to clarify any difficulties the husband may have. His comments or questions may reveal many of the attitudes which are likely to lead to difficulty for his wife.

It should be noted that the obstetrician and midwife have a primary responsibility to the mother, and that their concern with her is largely to ensure that she has her best chance of stability and security. If however, their discussion with the husband suggests he has major emotional problems or frank psychiatric illness himself, they should then advise him to seek help from his own practitioner. Many women will have difficult, obstinate, quick-tempered or stupid husbands, and many of these personality defects cannot be altered. Nevertheless, it is essential to know of their existence if the stresses on the patient are to be adequately assessed and if the total situation is to be managed aright.

Some immature husbands have relied on 'motherly' wives. These wives may be willing to 'mother' their husbands for a time, but the arrival of a real baby may lead to considerable stress. The husband may then feel rejected and, in turn, either reject his wife or be unable to give her the emotional support she needs. He may look for emotional support for himself elsewhere, perhaps returning to an earlier adjustment as 'one of the boys' or to find solace in alcohol. In either event, his wife will lose such support as he could have given.

Some women do lose their husbands—either temporarily as when a sailor goes to sea, or permanently by death. Some men desert their pregnant wives only to return once the child is born. This desertion may be complete or partial, as when the husband merely spends more time with his friends or on his sports or hobbies. We may speculate that such desertion is due to guilt over his sexual activities or simply loss of interest in someone who is no longer so attractive. Whatever the mechanism it is important to know whether or not the husband is able to give his wife both the material and the emotional support she needs.

Husbands who are closely identified with their wives tend to suffer with them. Some cultures allow for this in the rites of the couvade. In our culture, the husband's pangs of anxiety tend to be laughed at and are sometimes the subject of cartoons. Some attention to his anxiety however, will enable him to give more stability to his wife. Discussion and information will be of more value to both than tranquillizers, alcoholic or otherwise, for him alone.

The patient's mother

Almost all writers who have looked at the relationship between mother and daughter are agreed that it is one of the most important of all at the time of childbearing, and that any difficulties in the relationship may be revealed at that time. Most women feel a need for their mother's moral support and goodwill over their pregnancy and childbearing. Equally, those who have attained maturity feel that their ability to bear a child is a hallmark of adult life and are determined to have this achievement without recourse to assistance from their mother. It is inevitable that those women who are immature, over-dependent on their mothers, or have had previous emotional conflict in their relationship with their mother, will find that all the old difficulties recur during their own childbearing. For most women, of course, their most vital experience of the mother/child relationship is their own experience when they were a child in relation to their own mother. Many will have had further experience when their mother had further children. They may accept their mother's behaviour and attitudes as the normal ones in this situation and, in turn, repeat their mother's pattern. If, however, they have rejected their mother's standards, they may easily go to the other extreme in their own reactions. If all goes well, it is usually fairly easy for the patient's mother to remain a background figure. If there are difficulties it is all too common to find that this background figure now emerges and all the old conflicts and emotional difficulties recur. There is a particular risk in this situation that the patient's mother, in her attempts to help, will take over the patient's baby, in theory to lighten the latter's load. This should be avoided if possible since resentment is inevitable on the part of the patient. It is less satisfying for the patient's mother to take on the household chores, so that her daughter can give her entire attention to the infant, but there is no doubt that this is the preferable arrangement. Lastly, it is difficult for a mother who has any doubts about the wisdom of her daughter's choice to refrain from blaming the patient's husband for any difficulties her daughter has.

In-laws

The husband's parents also readily become involved in the emotional constellation surrounding childbirth. As in the case of the patient's mother, their emotional support is essential for harmony, but should there be difficulties it is likely that they will look for faults in their daughter-in-law and her family. Under the impact of psychiatric illness both sides of the family will tend to search their family tree, re-examine skeletons in the cupboard, and be prepared to find the fault in the other party. On the other hand, the baby, which can be such a disrupting influence can be unifying too, and many a family feud can be healed if both sides can be helped to understand the emotional problems involved, and the fact that any perpetuation of the conflict will harm the child.

The general practitioner

The chief difficulty for the general practitioner is in assessing the significance of symptoms, particularly early in the puerperium. Since major mental illness is relatively rare, but minor illness very common, his difficulty lies in deciding which one of the patients he sees will develop the major illness. In the course of a year the average general practitioner is not likely to see a major mental illness in the pueperium but will certainly see many tearful women, many who feel that for a time they cannot manage their child or household, and many who have insomnia or other psychiatric symptoms, any one of which could herald a major psychosis. It is very likely that in the course of a year he will see one or two patients whose history shows that there have been significant changes in their attitudes and competence since childbirth and they may have had significant psychiatric handicaps over many years. He will certainly want to know how such persistent handicaps could be prevented with modern methods of treatment and how he could predict the risk of such prolonged handicaps in the early stages of the illness. Since there is still some prejudice towards psychiatry, he may be reluctant to refer any but the most obvious case of mental illness for a psychiatric opinion, but will not wish to retain full responsibility for a patient who may create a major emotional incident in his practice. It is understandable therefore that the general practitioner will experience rather more anxiety in dealing with puerperal psychiatric symptoms than with a similar patient outside the puerperium. He will be further concerned since the majority of mothers in this country who require mental hospital admission will be unable to take their baby with them. Therefore, if admission becomes necessary he will have the further responsibility of advising on the baby's care and future. Like everyone else in this situation, he will fluctuate between a natural desire to keep mother and baby together and the fear that doing so will harm either or both.

The general practitioner will also face some uncertainty in

his prescribing. For example, the use of sedatives for the relief of anxiety will be contra-indicated, since the drowsy mother may be a danger to her child in the day and fail to attend to its needs by night. If she is breast-feeding, he may be uncertain which of the modern drugs, particularly the tranquilizers, are likely to be secreted in the milk in sufficient quantity to harm the child. It is almost traditional to take the baby off the breast when the mother shows any sort of nervous symptoms. This again is based on the theory that lactation is a 'strain', yet many a general practitioner must have found that by taking the child off the breast, he adds the problems of mixing feeds, maintaining an adequate temperature, and sterilization of bottles, to the anxious mother's other practical problems. Some women also resent advice which they feel frustrates their maternal instincts, though others may welcome it.

Another unfortunate situation may also lead to difficulties. Many women are no longer delivered by their own general practitioner. This means that for a vital time in her life, the patient is in the hands of another doctor. If the general practitioner has seen his patient through a satisfactory and placid pregnancy to find on her return from the maternity unit that he has a very anxious and unsettled patient, demanding frequent attention and reassurance, it will be easy for him to blame the maternity unit and overlook other significant factors in the situation. On the other hand, the general practitioner has some real advantages. If he has lived in a stable residential area for any length of time, he will know the family and background of his patients. He may even know the obstetric history of his present patient's mother and may know a great deal about the family attitudes and reactions to the stress of childbearing. This type of personal knowledge and first hand observation is of course denied to the obstetrician.

The obstetrician

Until very recent years, the obstetrician has tended to have a primary concern with the mechanics of labour rather than with the emotional component. There is no doubt that good obstetricians have always paid attention to their patient's emotional condition, though this attention was concealed beneath terms such as 'a good bedside manner'. In recent years increasing attention has been paid to the influence of the emotions at pregnancy, labour and the puerperium, and this influence was recognized at the First International Congress of Psychosomatic Medicine and Maternity held in Paris in 1962. Nevertheless, the vast majority of obstetricians have no specific psychiatric training and, like the general practitioner, will have the problem of picking out from among the mass of patients those few whose minor symptoms herald a major breakdown. They also have the additional handicap that they only see the patient during one episode of her life. Moreover, they may be completely misled by the emotional changes of pregnancy. Meeting a woman for the first time in the middle of pregnancy will give an unreliable guide to her true emotional stability. Many women are undoubtedly more stable at this time than at any other, even those who are usually timid or over-sensitive. The obstetrician may see the patient through a number of childbearing cycles, but this is unlikely unless the patient has a recurring physical disability as well, since the 'normal case' will be dealt with either by junior medical staff, who usually move from post to post, or by the midwife. It is difficult in this situation for the obstetrician to feel he is providing a continuing service and he must be tempted to hope that the early symptoms he sees in the maternity unit are merely a temporary matter and will be relieved by the patient's return home. Since the early symptoms of psychiatric disease fluctuate, so that between the time he is first notified of symptoms and the time he sees the patient they may have disappeared, the tendency to underestimate their significance is reinforced. Like the general practitioner, he will be reluctant to get the reputation of calling in a psychiatrist too soon. Nevertheless, it is to be hoped that he will not adopt the attitude of one obstetrician, who writes that he does not call in a psychiatrist to deal with delusions unless they fail to go away 'in the normal course of events'! A woman feels that she hands her life and that of her unborn child over to the obstetrician and this inevitably leads her to expect from him obvious personal concern and almost godlike infallibility. Since she is also particularly sensitive during childbirth and shortly after, she will readily over-react to remarks or attitudes which she feels are rejecting or critical. Subsequent difficulties with the child will be readily blamed either on herself or those taking care of her during these critical hours. Some remark, long since forgotten by the obstetrician may be treasured or resented by the patient for long periods or for life. Her management during labour and the first few days after childbirth set the scene for her love affair with her child and can easily make or mar this relationship.

Quite apart from the major illnesses, the evidence suggests that the way in which her emotions during childbearing are managed will have a prolonged effect on any woman's attitudes to the child, and to subsequent childbearing.

The ward sister and midwife

The ward sister probably has the most difficult task of all. She will be responsible for the care of many women whom she may never have seen before and may never see again after their few days on her ward. Even in the course of a week, she will only be in charge of a ward for a fifth of the total time available. The earliest signs of instability will often be noted by her or reported to her. She may become adept at assessing their immediate significance (and perhaps in suppressing them) but it is inevitable that she cannot know their long-term significance or the eventual outcome unless there be some dramatic incident. The midwife giving domiciliary care is in a much better position and it is significant that investigations have shown the majority of complaints made by women of their care during childbirth and the puerperium are made by those delivered in hospital, where in theory every convenience, skill and effort could be provided; but very few complaints are made by those delivered in their own homes. This finding may be relevant to my own observations that major psychoses develop very much more frequently in mothers delivered in a maternity unit than in mothers delivered at home.

Conclusions

It is obvious enough that the husband's attitudes can effect his wife's stability during childbearing. For example, some studies have shown that his presence will shorten the duration of labour. Equally, the attitudes and personality of the obstetrician or midwife can have obvious effect on the mother's emotional state. Medical students spend a considerable amount of time learning the exact mechanics of labour, both normal and abnormal, but are given relatively little guidance concerning the patient's emotional state, and even less about their own. Just as each mother brings her own attitudes, hopes and fears to childbearing, so the obstetrician and midwife bring theirs. For example, not all midwives are 'motherly' figures, some are frustrated spinsters who spend their lives seeing others achieve success in a sphere denied them. Nevertheless their contribution to the maternity services may be invaluable. Like all those involved in the situation they will play their part most effectively if there is awareness and understanding of their own problems.

It can be seen that the arrival of a baby creates a situation in which the anxiety of all participants may be increased for a variety of reasons. The relatives, physicians and nurses are all involved. As mentioned earlier, recourse to text-books will prove unsatisfactory for the doctor just as recourse to other families' solutions or the attitudes of the previous generation will be of little help to the particular family currently involved. It is essential for the doctors concerned to make an accurate assessment of all the factors in question. It is probably more important to take an accurate history in this situation than in any other. The history forms the basis not only for diagnosis but gives clues for management, and it is intended to discuss the history-taking in detail in the next chapter.

CHAPTER THREE
The History

It is essential to consider the psychiatric history at the first ante-natal interview. Just as enquiry will be made for the salient facts of previous physical health, so must some enquiry be made about the patient's mental health. It is essential that this should be done at the first interview and with the same practical approach as the enquiry about physical illness. If not, the patient may well feel that this part of her health is of no interest to her doctor or, alternatively, that he feels there is something disgraceful about it, and this will make her even more reluctant to discuss it on a further occasion. Nevertheless, because there is still considerable prejudice concerning mental illness, much more allowance must be made and more care taken in the phrasing of questions and in the attitude displayed by the physician.

A very brief outline of the major facts can be elicited in a matter of minutes at a first interview and possible relevant matters noted for further discussion; for example, the patient can be asked if her parents are alive and, if not, the cause of death. She can be asked about siblings and their health. In each case enquiry should be made in general terms of any history in close relatives of heart disease, chest condition, nervous breakdown, or other illness. The doctor should appear to be fairly casual, but should note any hesitant or vague answers for later clarification. If the patient was an only child it is often important to find out if she knows the reason for this. It is also important to clarify whether she was brought up by her own mother or adopted. Also in the first brief interview enquiry can be made about previous physical illness or nervous breakdown in herself and a general enquiry made about her personality and attitudes. Does she consider herself frail or robust? Does she consider herself of 'nervous temperament'? for example. This type of enquiry sets the scene for a more detailed assessment of the patient's background at a subsequent interview and will also make it clear to her that all aspects of her health are of equal interest.

During the interview, the physician should be concerned not merely with the factual answers as given, but also with the patient's emotional reactions. He should note whether she seems at ease or becomes restless and embarrassed by certain questions. He should note his own reactions as the interview progresses, since his own feelings towards the patient are often a guide to the patient's emotional state. The severe depressive almost always communicates her unhappiness, whereas the patient with schizophrenia frequently leads to an increasing feeling of perplexity in the interviewer. As far as is possible, the same person should see the patient at subsequent interviews. Whereas it is often irrelevant who tests the urine, there is no doubt that it matters very much to the patient who conducts interviews, and much of the possibility of understanding her and her difficulties would be thrown away if there is no continuity in this respect. The patient with emotional difficulties —and this of course applies to all women at some time—will feel a need for a continuing relationship with her physician, and this relationship cannot be transferred to another person. The patient does not have faith in doctors in general but in *her* doctor in particular.

Once the patient has confidence that she can talk freely, it is usually easy to obtain a full history quite quickly. Time spent in the early stages, however, will be saved over and over again. As mentioned in an earlier chapter it is important to check the facts of the history with some external observer, preferably the husband. During pregnancy and in the puerperium a woman's opinions are more coloured by her emotional state than at any other time.

The family history

It is obviously important to know if the patient's mother has
had any psychiatric illness. Some idea of her temperament will
be obtained indirectly from the patient's comments about her
but if these are insufficient, enquiry should be made to find out
if she was emotionally unstable, prudish, hard-hearted, over-
protective, or showed other conspicuous attitudes likely to
influence child-rearing. It is worth noting if the mother had
any kind of illness following childbirth. It will often be found
that 'milk fever', 'being run down' and similar terms cover a
psychiatric illness. The patient's mother may have been advised
to have no more children and the reasons for this are as likely
to be because of her psychiatric condition as any physical disturbance. Should the patient's mother have died, the age of the
patient at the time is relevant. If the death occurred soon after
childbirth and the precise cause is not known, suicide may be a
possibility and there may be a conspiracy of silence to conceal
the fact. The knowledge that her mother has died soon after
childbirth is likely to be a source of anxiety for any woman in
her own pregnancy. Girls who have been adopted or those who
have had many changes of home—whatever the reason—may
have considerable emotional insecurity as a result, however
mature their external appearance.

Similar enquiry should elicit the health and temperament of
the patient's father. In obtaining the history of both parents, it
will usually be easy to discover the relationship between them,
the stability of the home, and the emotional alignment of the
patient, if there have been parental quarrels. Much can be
learnt from the choice of expression. Girls who describe their
mothers as 'perfect' often show an over-dependency on their
mothers and a diffidence in asserting their own individuality.
This in turn is likely to make them fearful of the responsibility
of motherhood. Girls with 'perfect' fathers may be over-
dependent on their fathers, diffident about risking marriage
and may well alternate between idolizing their husbands and

finding the latter unable to live up to the idealized standard set by the father. They may try to adopt the same childlike role towards their husband and may feel this role threatened by the presence of a true baby in the house.

The patient's siblings, particularly her sisters, will give further clues, both about the inherited tendencies in the family as well as about the emotional constellation surrounding the patient's upbringing. Careful enquiry about the success of her sisters' marriages and the effects of childbearing will usually readily reveal any marked tendency to jealousy and may also bring out some of the family's traditions about child-rearing. Knowledge of the difficulties her sister has experienced in child-bearing may have almost as profound an effect upon the patient as the knowledge of her mother's difficulties.

Apart from specific enquiry about these close relatives—and in the present state of our knowledge these are the only specific enquiries necessary—it is always worth asking the patient if there is, in general terms, any family history of mental illness or abnormality. Not uncommonly it will be found that the patient does have some knowledge of a second cousin twice removed who became peculiar following childbirth and it may be of considerable importance to her to discuss the significance of such a history. As a fear of mental illness following childbirth is by no means uncommon, but is not as a rule readily admitted, it may be freely discussed if the opportunity is provided in this way. The fewer hidden anxieties the patient has within herself, and the fewer emotional barriers between her and her attendants, the smoother is the progress of pregnancy, confinement and puerperium likely to be.

Upbringing

The doctor will be interested in the patient's upbringing and early life because this will affect her attitudes towards child-birth. Considerable information about her parents and, in particular, her mother's treatment will have been revealed in the enquiry about the mother's health and relationship with her husband. There are some positions in the family however which are notorious for having a marked impact on the attitudes of any girl. For example, the eldest girl of a large family will certainly have extensive experience of the effects of childbirth and child-rearing on her mother's health and stability. It is very likely indeed that this eldest girl will find her own childhood curtailed because she was expected to accept responsibility for her younger siblings. Although this experience can be valuable, it is also common to find that these eldest girls resented the restrictions on their own pleasures as well as the inevitable limited affection from their mothers. In later life they may resent child-rearing, particularly if they marry someone who expects a large family, or if they have a large family because of their religious convictions.

The only child in a family will also have difficulties. Unless more distant relatives or neighbours are welcoming when they have a baby it is unlikely she will have much experience of the early days of baby life or of the practical problems of baby-rearing. The very fact that she is an only child will have its influence and she will certainly wonder why her own mother was unable or unwilling to have more. It is likely she had a great deal of attention and there is always the risk that she will have been over-protected. Inevitably, she will be more likely to expect similar attention and over-protection in the future from her husband, her doctors, her nurses, and may react with feelings of rejection and depression to the normal stresses and disappointments of everyday life. The youngest girl in the family often has the same difficulties as the only child. Youngest children are often idolized by their parents and also supported and protected by the elder siblings. This degree of emotional support may never be available again later in life.

Some enquiry should be made about the patient's previous attitudes and behaviour. For example, it is worth noting whether her school adjustment was easy or not and whether she had much time off for minor ill-health. Her ability to make friends readily and her hobbies and interests may be pointers to her personality. It is all too common, however, to find that patients will paint a picture of their previous personality which is much too dependent on their present emotional state. Nevertheless, school adjustment and the work record will almost certainly give a clue to the patient's intelligence level and also her level of social aspiration. Similarly, the school record and work record, including the reasons for changing jobs will usually pick out the patient with any previous difficulties in her relationship with other people, particularly with those in authority.

The details of the patient's sexual history will usually be obtained at more than one interview. A few women will talk freely and readily but, even in 1967, the majority still feel this part of their life is more private than most other aspects. Some idea of her probable attitudes will be obtained when discussing her mother and, in particular, whether her mother was prudish or otherwise. It is often easy to begin with the facts of menstruation, and prior instruction about its onset, which is almost always linked with previous information about sexual activities. Discussion of this will often reveal the patient's own feeling towards herself as a woman and whether she feels pride and pleasure in her femininity or feels it to be in some way a disadvantage. Her attitude towards her own sexual reactions may be very complicated and many women find it difficult to verbalize. Moreover, the attitude may change very considerably, even for example, during the course of the monthly cycle, when some women's acceptance of their own femininity may change from obvious pleasure to repugnance. Changes in the emotional state during the pre-menstrual phase often give a very useful guide to the patient's emotional stability under the stress of hormonal changes and specific enquiry about this should always be made.

The patient's choice of husband is often revealing. Apart from the obvious case in which an immature and father-dependent girl marries a man twenty years older than herself, there are many more subtle situations which, nevertheless, reveal the patient's problems or attitudes. The woman who is so fearful of masculine domination that she marries an inadequate husband, the woman who is prudish and inhibited and therefore marries a man as shy and diffident as herself, or the woman who marries the first man who is willing, in order to get away from a disturbed home, are all obvious examples of relationships where emotional repercussions are inevitable if she begins to bear children.

Some general enquiry about sexual activities and satisfactions in the marriage should be made. Here again, it is more important to make the woman feel at ease in the discussion and to leave her with the feeling that these problems *can* be ventilated, rather than to try and pry for details, particularly early in the doctor/patient relationship. An insistence on early confidence may merely make the patient deny all her difficulties and, once having committed herself to the opinion that her marriage is perfect, it will be more difficult for her to discuss the true state of affairs at a later date.

The most careful enquiry of all should be directed to the history surrounding any previous pregnancy. As a rule, women will talk quite freely on this subject and it is therefore worthwhile obtaining some detailed information. Enquiry should be made for the emotional reactions throughout pregnancy, for any specific symptoms at that time, for the emotional state before, during, and after labour, and the woman's opinions on how her confinement was conducted. The emotional repercussions of childbearing go on for months after the event; it is important to know how soon after childbirth the woman felt really well and whether she was aware of any changes in her own personality or attitudes as a whole. Repeated minor illness, 'investigations', or prolonged 'tiredness', difficulties in lactation, or lack of feeling for the baby and difficulties in childrearing, are often clear pointers to emotional problems. As with the other parts of the history, this part too must be checked with the husband, who may be more aware of personality changes in his wife following childbearing than she is herself.

It may seem that obtaining a history in the detail outlined here will be very time-consuming. In practice, however, all the details mentioned could be obtained from conversations taking place during the usual antenatal examinations. When some physical examinations are being made, checks on the position of the foetus, or similar routine care is being conducted, some of the time should be given over to enquiry into the psychiatric history. Provided some notes are taken, so that gaps in the history can be filled in at later interviews, it is unlikely that much more time will be needed in obtaining a full and detailed psychiatric history than would be given to the woman in any case. Moreover, the obstetrician or midwife will then have a much clearer picture of the type of person they will be caring for, her particular problems, her particular anxieties, her particular hopes and fears. Such knowledge must influence the attitudes of those around her and make it much more likely that they will automatically make the right adjustment to their own attitudes when this is necessary.

Much has been written in the popular, as well as medical, press about 'father figures' and 'mother figures'. There is no doubt that people tend to react towards their seniors, particularly those in authority, in a way which shows how they learnt to react in their early life. The man who had a stern father may tend to be over-anxious in the presence of a stern employer. A woman brought up by a doting mother may come to expect similar over-concern from older women in her adult life. Similarly, a woman who has been rejected by her own mother may well come to expect rejection on the part of women who are normally expected to be motherly or protective. This, like all human relationships, is a two-way affair. The over-dependent woman will appear immature and will tend to respond to an older woman who is willing to 'mother' her. An older woman who has had no children of her own may tend to respond to the need for 'mothering' in another person. The position is complicated by the fact that some children conform closely to their parents' standards, while others reject them and may even go to the opposite extreme. The tendency to react to other people in a way which has been determined by early life experiences is of vital importance in all human relationships and is particularly applicable in the situation at childbirth. It is not enough, however, to say that because a woman is dependent on her physician she will look on him as a father figure and may react towards him in a way which may reflect her relationship with her father, nor that she reacts towards the midwife in a way which will reflect her early response to her own mother. Obviously, a woman in her forties having her fifth child is unlikely to feel that a young houseman in his twenties and of limited experience is a 'father figure'. Nevertheless, if the patient's reactions to those around her at the time of childbirth are to be understood some knowledge of her early life and reaction to her parental figures should be known. Similarly, the general practitioner, obstetrician or midwife should know something of their own personality and of the sort of response they are likely to evoke in the woman under their care.

Present stress

The patient will have inherited a nervous system with a wide variety of potential responses to the environment. This responsiveness will have been modified by her upbringing and previous experience. It is usual to find, however, that in all mental illnesses there are some present stresses which have precipitated the actual symptoms. Pregnancy, childbirth, and child-rearing are stresses for any woman. There are some particular factors, however, which do require further consideration.

The patient's marital status is obviously relevant. Throughout the animal kingdom it is usual to find that where there is a consistent relationship between male and female, the former provides defence, food and shelter for the family. In the human, the husband's functions are essentially the same. The woman's anxiety, therefore, will be the greater if her husband has personality inadequacies which make him rely on her rather than the reverse. Similarly, if he is incompetent at work or unable to provide financial security her anxieties will be increased. Lastly, and this factor is easily overlooked, women need a secure 'nest' as a background for childbearing. Common observation will show that in the animal kingdom disturbance of the mother shortly after giving birth may lead to the offspring being abandoned. There is clinical evidence to support the opinion that a woman should be settled in her home during pregnancy and should not have a change of household in the early months after childbirth. Sometimes an ambitious and kind hearted husband may plan a new home for his wife and move into it when the baby arrives. From the point of view of the woman's emotional state this is the worst possible time for a change of house, unless her present accommodation is grossly unsatisfactory. Any change should be made outside pregnancy and the puerperium, if possible. If a change has to be made it should be arranged in the early stages of pregnancy or left until the child has been weaned. Unfortunately, of course, the husband's work may compel him to make a move at a time which is quite inconvenient for his wife. The actual housing conditions are of *relatively* little importance provided the patient feels 'at home'. A slum dweller accustomed to slum conditions may feel more secure in this background than if suddenly moved to a new and unfamiliar flat, even if it has all the modern conveniences.

Other children in the household place an emotional strain on the mother who may try too hard to share her affections and endeavour to give just as much care to the older children when the new baby has arrived. It is one of the functions of the father and other relatives to supply some of the emotional needs of the toddlers and older children, so that the mother is able to concentrate on the baby and give it the basic security it needs. Illness in the husband or other children, or serious difficulty in the relationships with them, will add to the mother's burdens.

Cultural problems are becoming more common. In one extreme example, a husband and wife have been encountered who did not speak each other's language, and had no common communication other than through signs. Since both came from overseas and spoke no English it is not surprising that they had become isolated in a London suburb, and both presented psychiatric symptoms. In lesser degree, however, cultural problems may be present which do not appear at first sight. For example, the country girl living in a town flat, or a Cockney girl living in the country, may both feel out of place, find it difficult to develop a social life and have far more emotional stress than might otherwise be expected. Under present conditions a considerable number of women have now married outside their own culture. This particularly applies to immigrants and visiting students, and the severity of the problem may be completely overlooked in the antenatal clinic unless some enquiry is made. Since it is likely that a woman marrying outside her own culture would have been advised against this, she is disposed to deny all difficulties rather than admit a mistake.

It is hardly necessary to point out that unmarried mothers will always have emotional problems, even if they have the full support of their family. Similarly, the woman who is abandoned by her husband and left to give birth and bring up his child will experience stress over the years.

For many years it was common to assume that physical illness must act as a precipitant of psychiatric disorders. More recently, however, it has become apparent that although the physical illnesses may be accompanied by toxic confusional states they do not commonly precipitate functional psychiatric conditions.

There is no clear relationship, for example, between toxaemia in pregnancy and any functional psychiatric disease in the puerperium. Similarly there is no close relationship between a difficult labour and subsequent depressive reaction. Most careful studies which have used control groups have shown that other factors are more important.

The stress of labour

It is quite striking that acute breakdowns rarely develop under the immediate stress of giving birth; even the dramatic schizophrenic illnesses usually develop some days later. Equally, it is true that the woman's normal emotional state—and particularly her emotional state during pregnancy—are no guide to her actual comportment during the labour. Many 'highly-strung' women have quick and easy labours and show relatively little emotional distress. It is more common to find that the middle-class housewife, who has learnt too well to control her feelings, finds this self-control a disadvantage during labour and may surprise her attendants when she reveals the depth of her distress. It is this type of mother who may express the greatest fear, rage and anger, which has probably led to some of the reports which suggest that such feelings are universal, but sometimes concealed. Childbirth is a process in which there needs to be harmony between the physical and emotional state, and a woman should be able to allow her feelings, as well as her muscles, free expression, and not the excessive control too commonly found in women who have had a restrictive upbringing.

The emotional atmosphere around the woman who is giving birth is as important as the physical care. Just as the obstetrician will wish to avoid insanitary conditions, so he will wish to avoid emotional insecurity. It has been said with truth, that physical security lies in the hospital, but emotional security in the home. Admission to hospital for childbirth is in itself an admission that the process is potentially dangerous, and may serve to confirm some women's fears. We must therefore consider the anxieties which the hospital itself can engender.

The hospital buildings are often strange and unfamiliar. Their sights, sounds and smells are frequently associated with illness and tragedy. The mother's previous experience may have been a miserable and grisly one when she had her tonsils removed twenty years previously. Under present conditions it is not unknown for a woman to be admitted to a hospital she has never seen before in her life. Quite apart from such an extreme example, it is clear that hospital admission is an emotional stress for every woman. Apart from ignorance of the building and its functions, she may not know any of her attendants. She may well find that the doctor or midwife who delivers her was not the one she saw in the antenatal clinic. A woman needs to have full confidence in her attendant at this time and this is hardly possible if this is their first acquaintance. Every effort should be made to ensure that a woman having a hospital confinement does know the bare essentials of the building and its rooms and has at least met and can recognize those who will deliver her.

The obstetrician will assess the relative risks of home confinement compared with hospital confinement in the presence of any physical disability and should consider the emotional risks in exactly the same way. Some women's anxiety might well indicate that a hospital confinement would be preferable. If, for example, she had a specific fear of haemorrhage following childbirth, perhaps because a friend or relative had suffered from this, a hospital confinement might help to relieve this fear. On the other hand, fears of germs and contamination are quite common and the more intelligent woman may know of the risks of hospital infections, in which case a home confinement would be preferable. In every case, however, it is essential that the emotional state should receive the same consideration as the physical state in reaching a decision. There is no advantage for the patient in escaping a physical complication, merely to have her life made miserable by emotional problems.

The young mother has particular difficulties in hospital once her baby is born. It will be more difficult for her to be spontaneous in her reaction to her own child with strangers present. She will be distressed by hearing other babies cry, and wondering if it is hers. If her own child cries she may wonder if she should attend to its needs or wait for the nurse to advise. Some mothers feel that the baby is not really theirs until they get home and have it to themselves. The unfamiliarity of hospital life, the presence of strangers, an enforced routine, and the many doubts, are all adverse factors which militate against the smooth development of the love affair with her baby.

Relevance of factors in the history

The details of the history, together with the patient's response to discussion and enquiry will give many clues to her probable reaction under stress. Particular consideration must be given to any history of previous mental illness. In the case of the neuroses these illnesses are more common in the younger mother and following the first child, and may not recur with subsequent children even if the physical conditions are less satisfactory than previously. The severe neuroses with persistent conflicts usually lead to a limitation of further child-bearing. It is usual of course to find that the *type* of neurotic reaction is likely to be repeated should the patient's adjustment begin to fail. The other class of patient where neurotic symptoms may appear is in the woman who married late, or started child-bearing late in life. In general the younger woman is more emotionally labile and will tend to adjust more rapidly to a new situation. In the older woman this lability has been lost and she may find the adaptation to the new relationship and further responsibility very difficult.

A previous history of depression is particularly hard to evaluate. Minor degrees of depression are extremely common but, if there is a history of severe (psychotic) depression following a first child, there is a one in four likelihood that a similar illness will develop following subsequent childbearing. In general the likelihood of severe depressions becomes greater with advancing age. A history of two previous depressive episodes would make a further depression following additional childbearing much more probable. There is no absolute rule in this situation, and it is quite possible for a woman who has had two severe depressions to have a further child and remain emotionally stable. On the other hand, the history is a better guide than the patient's emotional state during pregnancy. Many women who are more stable and competent than usual during pregnancy may have severe depressive symptoms a few months after the birth of the baby.

A previous history of schizophrenia is of more ominous import. If the patient has had a schizophrenic illness at any time in her life it is likely that the stress of childbearing will lead to a relapse at some time in the months following childbirth. A previous history of schizophrenia in the puerperium does not necessarily carry greater weight than schizophrenia at some other time. It is particularly important to remember that patients who have had schizophrenia do tend to be relatively well during pregnancy, and many of them who are aware of this, welcome childbearing. Their lack of insight will prevent them from making an adequate assessment of their illness in the puerperium. It is probable that the idea that women with schizophrenia were infertile was a result of statistics taken from a limited population. Many women with this disease seem to conceive with ease. This is becoming of increasing importance now that the illness can be treated with greater success, in that many more women who have had schizophrenia are living in the community instead of being isolated in mental hospitals.

A previous history of organic reaction, for example, a delirium, is of little relevance other than the anxiety it may cause the patient who will fear a repetition. Obviously, such a reaction is only likely to recur if the physical illness causing it is also likely to recur, and presumably steps can be taken to prevent this. It is likely, however, that the patient who has had one delirious reaction is more likely to react with delirium under similar stress than other members of the population.

CHAPTER FOUR

Common Emotional Reactions in Pregnancy and the Puerperium

Although the patient's own personality will influence to a marked degree the course of her pregnancy and subsequent child-rearing, some allowance must also be made for the influence these events have upon the patient's own reactions, in particular her emotional lability. It is a commonplace that women show more emotional instability at times when there are major changes in hormone levels, for example, at puberty, in the pre-menstrual phase, or at the menopause. Very much greater changes in the hormone levels occur during pregnancy and the puerperium. It should not be surprising therefore to find significant alterations in mood to correspond with this.

The first three months of pregnancy are characterized by considerable emotional lability with an undercurrent of anxiety. It is common to find that even placid women show some irritability or uneasiness at this time. Those women who are normally emotionally unstable are likely to show this to a greater degree. It is during the first three months that many women will show obvious ambivalence towards the foetus. They may bewilder their husbands by appearing delighted with the pregnancy on one day and then to bewail their fate the next. It is at this time that stresses in the marriage may become apparent. Any symptoms from the pregnancy may be exaggerated and the husband's feelings tested by his solicitude for the sufferer. It is probable that changes in hormone level underlie both the morning sickness and the various alterations in choice of food. Many women develop some minor craving or aversion and will test their husband's affection by his willingness to provide the dainty of their choice. This emotional lability has some advantages. For example, the majority of women withstand the loss of the foetus in the first three months with the minimum of emotional repercussion. The ambivalence in their attitude enables them to make a rapid adjustment to the loss.

The middle three months of pregnancy are usually characterized by an increased emotional stability and frequently with an apparent increase in self-confidence and drive. This is the phase in which women 'make their nest', begin to organize their household, and the early ambivalence to the child disappears. Many women are aware of feeling healthier and more stable at this time than at any other time in their lives. They present the classical picture of 'blooming health' both physical and emotional. The earlier nausea subsides and the woman becomes concerned with the practical details of her own and the baby's future. She will often surprise her husband by appearing to have matured and to show a competence and determination he had never suspected. This can have its repercussions if an inadequate husband learns to lean too heavily on his wife, or a rigid one to thwart her initiative. From the fourth month onwards, however, abortion or miscarriage is likely to be felt by the woman as a true loss of a child and more serious emotional repercussions are then possible.

The last three months of pregnancy are characterized by an increase in lethargy, both physical and emotional. There is also an undercurrent of anxiety as the day for labour approaches. The sluggishness usually means that the woman begins to make increasing demands on her husband to manage the practical realities of day to day affairs. In the last few weeks of pregnancy any fears the patient has with regard to her safety or the well-being of her child will gradually appear. It is at this time that the first warning of an eventual psychiatric breakdown may be given. Many stable women, however, will need some reassurance about their physical safety and the normality of their child as far as it can be assessed. All woman must know that there is a risk of death in childbirth however small that risk is under present conditions. Many of them have other fears added by misguided friends or old wives' tales, or from their own previous unhappy experience. The more these fears can be relieved, the less emotional stress the mother will experience when her time comes. She will however only reveal her fears if she has some confidence in her attendant and this is yet another reason why some continuity in the relationship between the mother and midwife or obstetrician is essential.

Many women notice that on the day the baby actually arrives they experience a curious calm and detachment once they are aware that childbirth is imminent. In another large group however there is the opposite reaction. Such women feel a sudden urge to activity and will undertake physically exacting tasks which, on reflection, they would know are quite inappropriate. For example, one will clean out her cupboards or pantry, another will start a small-scale spring-clean, yet a third who has ample domestic help, will scrub her own floors for the first time perhaps in years. It is tempting to assume that some hormonal or neuronal impulse which leads to the increased activity in the uterus has led to an increase in the woman's general activity. It may well be, however, that once the woman is aware of the imminence of childbirth she feels a desperate need to complete any undone tasks, lest she be unable to complete them in the future. Whatever the reason, some women are aware that this sudden spurt of activity is clear warning that the baby is due.

Once labour is under way most women become increasingly pre-occupied with themselves and in some measure detached from their surroundings. This detachment however is selective and it is notorious that a woman who appears oblivious to all around her while concentrating on the contractions of her uterus may pick up a casual remark from a bystander and take obvious offence or pleasure when neither was intended. In general, childbirth tends to be easier in the younger patient. It is often easier in those women who seem able to give free rein or expression to their feelings, whereas the inhibited and over-controlled suburban housewife may have an over-inhibited and prolonged labour. Many 'nervous', histrionic and emotionally labile women who feared a prolonged labour, often have a short and easy one; whereas the apparently composed and perhaps over-confident suburban housewife may take many hours before she can allow her uterus to take over control of proceedings. Labour is hard work and is most readily and satisfactorily accomplished if the woman's emotions are fully co-ordinated with her physical activities. Those who find their lives restricted by anxieties and fears may find their labour similarly affected.

Women's attitudes and reactions to the whole process of childbirth vary considerably and are undoubtedly deeply rooted in their personality, upbringing and culture. For some it is nothing but a cruel ordeal through which they have to pass to acquire their baby. For others the whole process is like some vast excretion. Yet others can feel the same sort of excitement and ecstasy as in an orgasm. Depending on her total attitude and the experience itself, so will her feelings be affected at the actual moment of birth. For some it is indeed a moment of great joy, for others there is the feeling of reward for work accomplished. For many, perhaps the majority, there is an immense feeling of relief. As soon as the baby has actually arrived it is almost universal to find the woman wishes to see it. One of the great fears which lie dormant in every woman is the fear that she will give birth to a deformed child. Only by seeing her own new-born in its entirety can she be assured that this particular child is indeed normal.

Many women who have anaesthetics never experience the actual moment when their child is born. Some of these women will merely express relief that what might have been a painful process has been reasonably comfortable. Others however will feel that they have failed to experience a vital part of the whole proceedings and may, curiously enough, feel some resentment towards those who, however well-meaning, deprived them in this way.

Immediately the child is born the mother is conscious of a wish to see it and handle it for herself. There is always a moment of anxiety during which she will wish to be reassured that the child is normal, and has no deformity or congenital abnormality. She is also concerned as to its sex. Some women feel strongly about the sex of their child and in some families there may be considerable emotional need for a child of one sex. Traditionally women want a boy, but this is not always the case. There are instances where some women have a strong desire for a girl. Sometimes the reasons for these choices are practical and obvious to all, for the woman who already has three of one sex may wish the fourth to be different. Sometimes of course the need for a child of a particular sex is deeply rooted in past experiences, past hopes and past fears. Occasionally the failure to have the child of the desired sex may lead to considerable disappointment in the young mother and she may for a long period resent the child and the disappointment it caused her. Much more commonly, however, the mother who has expressed a strong desire for one sex is nevertheless delighted with the baby she has and rapidly adjusts to the situation. Occasionally the woman herself may be happy to have a child of either sex, but her husband, for a variety of reasons, may strongly desire one particular sex, usually a boy. The patient may find it difficult to tolerate her husband's disappointment and may feel she has failed him, even though it was clearly not her fault.

After her first handling of her own child and the reassurance this gives her, most women need sleep. Frequently sleep comes easily but occasionally mothers find that the stress and excitement of labour leave them with a persistent feeling of tension. Just as they begin to fall asleep memories of labour come into their mind and they wake again, beginning to relive the episode. If this is associated with some abdominal discomfort, as is not uncommon, sleep may be spoilt for several nights. This situation should not be allowed to continue and it is a clear indication for adequate sedation.

Many women find that a few days following childbirth they feel an unexpected degree of depression. All the joyful expectation seems to disappear and they are left with a feeling of misery and an unexpectedly gloomy outlook. Their husband on visiting may find them tearful and disinterested either in the baby or his own news. This reaction has been sufficiently common to acquire the popular name of the 'four-day blues'. It is likely that this has many causes. It is worth noting that it is more common following a hospital confinement than one at home. It may well be associated with some of the frustration and boredom of hospital life. It may partly be a reflection of physiological changes, as the great drop in hormone levels occurs in the first few days following birth. It may also reflect a change in the woman's mood from one of increasing anticipation during late pregnancy to a gradual awareness, now the child is born, that not only does she have the pleasure and satisfaction of motherhood but also the chores and extra responsibility and limitation on her own satisfactions too. It has also been suggested that women have a true sense of loss once the child is born, in that it is no longer completely one with themselves.

Quite apart from the 'four-day blues', most women notice that during the first week after childbirth they are emotionally labile. They may become readily excited, easily pleased, easily disappointed. They may overact to trivial comments which can be taken too seriously. They may take to heart a casual remark and, equally, be exceedingly pleased with small praise. The chief focus of their attention is the baby. This emotional lability is probably a necessary emotional basis for falling in love with the new-born child. Certainly, to the outside observer, a somewhat volatile and emotional young mother seems to find it easier to fall in love with her babe than her more staid and inhibited sister. Maternal drives are partly inherited and developed on an instinctual basis. They must be conditioned by the mother's upbringing and also by the situation she finds herself in immediately after childbirth. There is no doubt she will fall in love with her baby and make a more satisfactory relationship with it, if she can do so in a place of security where she can obtain privacy and also emotional support. It is essential that she should feel approved and loved and what she is doing is right. She will be particularly sensitive to criticism or to any evidence of disapproval. It is very difficult in the hospital setting for a young mother to obtain these necessities in the relationship with her baby. It is not easy to give her privacy. It is not easy to give her the feeling that she is of the greatest importance and that those around her feel nothing but affection for her. Moreover, in the busy hospital scene, changes of staff, frequent movements, comings and goings, all create an atmosphere which militates against a feeling of security.

Each mother/baby relationship is unique and is formed between this particular mother and this particular baby. Each must learn to react and adjust to the other. It is quite impossible for this relationship to be learnt from books or to be obtained by instruction from others. Some confidence in the practical aspects can be obtained by watching others but each woman must find a way that satisfies *her*. For some women a routine by which the baby is fed regularly, cuddled regularly, and tended regularly, is for them satisfactory and, for this reason, their baby is likely to adjust to this situation. For another woman, feeding by demand and attention given when apparently needed will satisfy her, and probably lead to the best adjustment between her and her child. Again, it is extremely difficult within a hospital setting to let each mother develop her own relationship. A mother needs to feel that it really is her baby for which she has laboured. In hospital, unless there is a very good rooming-in system, it is all too easy to feel that the baby belongs to the nurses until she can actually get it home. It is common to hear of increasing anxiety, tension and frustration in mothers lying in maternity wards. They may lie and hear babies crying and become increasingly anxious and tense. They may be unsure whether to attend to the child, and they describe lying sweating, with milk streaming from their breasts, in a state of extreme frustration. It is not surprising to find therefore that beneath the apparent calm of many women in a maternity ward there lies considerable frustration and anxiety, and much of this may be unloaded on the husband at his visits. It is common to find considerable pressure is put on husbands to take their wives home, even though it is equally well known that once at home, mothers may have other pressures and family responsibilities thrust upon them.

Some women, who are frequently looked on as 'good' mothers, behave very well in the maternity unit and obey any instructions implicitly. These women are frequently somewhat immature, have been 'good' girls at home and frequently 'good' wives. They are able to function efficiently while receiving supervision, guidance and instruction, and when somebody else takes full responsibility. These mothers may break down rapidly on return home, when they find their husband has gone to work and they are left with the full responsibility for the baby as well as the daily routine, quite on their own. Panic attacks, phobic symptoms, weeping, and other neurotic reactions, are common in this sort of patient shortly after leaving hospital. These women have often had a 'roses round the door' outlook on marriage and child-rearing and the practical realities of the day-to-day chores, hard work, and inconvenience comes as a considerable shock and disappointment to them.

Among the other common reactions, it is essential to mention the difficulties which will be experienced if the mother either loses her baby at birth or, alternatively, has an abnormal child. Clearly, if she loses her child at birth or soon after, some degree of depression is inevitable. It is important to remember that such a reaction is normal, to be expected and, indeed, a period of mourning is essential for the woman's future emotional health. She should not be urged to forget the child or to have another one to replace it. No woman should be urged to have a child to replace the one she has lost. If she does, it is very likely indeed that she will expect too much of this child and will expect it to make up for all the suffering she had as a result of the loss of the first. This will almost certainly spoil the relationship from the beginning. A woman should have a baby because she wants that particular child, not merely one to replace another. If, therefore, the patient loses her child, tears, unhappiness and clear depression are to be accepted as normal reactions. It is particularly hard on such women to stay in hospital and see other mothers enjoying the fruits of their labours. It is often kinder to remove such a mother to a gynaeco-logical ward for a few days before going home.

In the case of a mother who has an abnormal child, emotional repercussions are equally inevitable. Again, it is probably better that she should express her regret and grief forthwith. It is essential to know the sort of patient with whom one is dealing and the sort of attitude she is likely to adopt. To impart the knowledge of abnormality is a very delicate task indeed which should normally be left to the consultant, general practitioner, or other senior physician making the diagnosis. It should always be done with care and understanding. Most women will experience some feeling of loss and will mourn the child they had hoped for but will now never have. Moreover, the child they have with its abnormality or deformity is a constant reminder to them of their disappointment. Nevertheless, partly because of the emotional lability during the first few days after childbirth, most women will feel strong maternal feelings to-wards the child, however deformed. Indeed, it is notorious that many women will lavish an excess of care on the most abnormal of their children even to the extent of neglecting others. It may be more difficult for the husband to accept the abnormality in the family than it is for the mother. It is equally important to help the parents to understand the causes of any abnormality. If there is any possibility of an inherited defect, the risks to further children should be explained. If, on the other hand, it is clearly due to some incident during labour this too should be explained, and whether or not it is likely to recur in the future. As might be expected, most women can cope better with a real and practical difficulty than with some un-known fear. It is important, before the mother leaves hospital, that she should have some idea of the outlook for her child and the sort of care it may need, the sort of progress it is likely to make, and of the part she and the doctors will have to play in the rearing. It may well be that the mother may need to stay in the maternity unit for a longer period if her child is abnormal, not only because of the difficulties there may be in the physical rearing of the child, but to give her sufficient time to make an emotional adjustment to it. Obviously, it is important to ensure that the patient has an introduction to the paediatric or other services which may be involved in any further treatment programme.

Lastly, we must consider the difficulties of the young mother who will be unable to rear her child. Under present conditions, many women have illegitimate babies and, for a variety of social reasons, decide they cannot bring the child up themselves. Many such women can make a sound decision on the question of adoption during the pregnancy, but certainly not all are able to do so. In particular, those with mental illness, psychopathy, or subnormality, may have difficulties. Occasionally, unfortunately, the very woman who is the least suitable to bring up the child and who is very likely indeed to become more unstable following childbirth, will be the one who tries to insist on retaining the child. This insistence may be part of her mental illness. For example, a patient with schizophrenia, who had been under treatment for many years, became pregnant as a result of an escapade following absconding from a mental hospital. The pregnancy was not discovered for five months and it was felt that, at this point, termination was unwise and carried greater risks than allowing it to continue. Although obviously psychotic throughout the pregnancy, she nevertheless insisted that she wished to keep the child once born and believed herself quite able to support herself and manage the child.

It is important that the woman should be given every opportunity to make her own decision about her ability to care for her child. On the other hand, it is sometimes necessary as in the case quoted, to use considerable persuasion if it is clear it is impossible for the patient to carry out her plans.

There has been too little investigation into the problem posed by early separation of mother and baby, from the point of view

of the mother. Some women like to give their child some attention during the first week of its life, even if they then lose it to
be fostered or adopted. Other women are well aware of the
fact that even a week's contact with the child will produce
intense maternal drives which will lead to considerable depression and emotional repercussions when the child is taken away.
There is good evidence to suggest that it is often better for the
mother and baby to be separated immediately after birth,
rather than allow contact for ten days, which is considered in
some maternity units. Any mother should be reassured that
her child is normal, if it is indeed the case, and it is probably
wise to allow her to see it so that there can be no possible doubt
about its physical normality. Once, however, she has begun to
handle it or feed it, maternal links and drives are undoubtedly
aroused and subsequent separation proves the harder. Obviously,
if there is some doubt about whether the woman will keep her
child, she should be given every opportunity and support.
Where, however, there is no future for the relationship it is
cruel to prolong it any longer than is strictly necessary.

CHAPTER FIVE

The Neuroses

Neurotic reactions are much more frequent than psychotic illnesses. Some minor neurotic *symptoms* not severe enough to justify a formal diagnosis are likely with the majority of mothers at some time during pregnancy or the puerperium. In the overt illness a family history of the condition is common, particularly in the obsessional states. Similarly, there is often a family history of personality traits predisposing to neurosis and, here again, the obsessional personality is likely to recur in succeeding generations. It has proved singularly difficult, even with carefully planned research, to show whether these personality traits are indeed inherited or acquired as a result of living within the family.

The neurotic illnesses are often regarded as minor, but in severe degree can prove just as much a handicap as the most florid psychosis. Although it is easy to point to the disturbance caused in a family by a psychotic member, the emotional distress caused by a patient with severe neurosis may be just as devastating. There is some evidence to suggest that the children of parents with obsessional traits or obsessional illnesses are more likely to be disturbed than the children of parents with a frank psychosis. It is difficult enough to try and draw a precise line between personality defects and the onset of a psychosis. It is even more difficult to draw the line between the normal reactions of a personality under stress and the development of neurotic symptoms, particularly in a person who has shown for many years a poor adjustment to the environment. It is often easier to describe a patient's condition in terms of the symptoms, the previous personality and current stress, rather than give a brief but unhelpful diagnosis. For example, a diagnosis of 'anxiety state' is of limited value, but the description of 'tension with anorexia in an immature and over-dependent patient who feels threatened by the responsibility of her baby' gives a much better picture of the problem, as well as providing some clue to the correct approach for treatment.

Neurotic symptoms tend to be most common in late adolescence and early adult life. They are therefore more common with first babies and the fact that the patient has had a neurosis after her first child has very little predictive value for her response after a second child. The patient may well have matured considerably and the knowledge that she has successfully reared one infant should give her confidence with her second. Therefore, the neurotic reactions tend to become less frequent as the patient becomes older. Some severe neuroses, particularly if they are associated with such symptoms as frigidity, tend inevitably to prevent further childbearing. An exception to the tendency for neurotic reactions to become less frequent in the older patient is in the case of a woman who has her first child relatively late in life. Some women who have developed a set pattern of life and then have a baby, either in a late marriage or unexpectedly after many years of marriage, may find it difficult to adjust to the total change in routine which a baby demands.

Most psychiatrists would accept that inheritance plays a limited part in the development of neurotic illness but that the patient's upbringing and family constellation play a very considerable role. Certainly in the neurotic illnesses the patient may reveal attitudes towards her own body, her own child, or her marital relationship, which are clearly related to her past life experience. It is even more important therefore to ensure that the family as a whole is considered in the treatment programme, and particular care should be taken in the management of any relationship with her own parents. If, as not uncommonly happens, the patient is still living under the parental roof, the correct management of this situation may be more important than any other aspect of the patient's care.

We shall consider the individual neuroses and their symptomatology to enable a distinction to be made between these and the early symptoms of the psychotic illness.

Anxiety states

These are probably the commonest of all the neurotic illnesses and present with a wide variety of symptoms. Usually the patient complains of feeling anxious and tending to over-respond to small stimuli. She may be aware of irritability and a general emotional lability. She often finds it difficult to get to sleep because the problems of the day go round in her mind. Once asleep, she sleeps lightly, is prone to nightmares and finds that this sleep pattern, particularly if aggravated by the baby's wakefulness, makes her even more irritable and unsettled in the day. The onset is usually associated with somatic symptoms and these may form the primary complaints. She may complain of tension, muscular pains or tremors, palpitations, 'butterflies in the stomach', frequency of micturition, or a wide variety of similar symptoms. Some patients will recognize that these are 'nervous' and related to their own emotional state, but insight is by no means universal and some patients will go from doctor to doctor with the same physical symptom, trying to find one who will discover at least some minimal organic lesion to account for it. Phobic symptoms usually develop on a basis of anxiety.

The relationship with the baby frequently shows these classical symptoms. The patient is over-solicitious and over-anxious, but her patience short-lived. She is usually willing to blame the child for her condition and willing to accept some-one's offer to take the child from her 'to give her a rest'. This temporary expedient frequently leads to long-term problems, especially if it is the patient's own mother who takes the child, or some other relative who might develop a strong feeling for the infant. If given an opportunity for a discussion of their feelings, these patients will often develop insight very quickly and readily admit their frustration and resentment towards the child. Insight easily acquired does not necessarily alter the patient's feelings or her inadequacy. It is a common finding that her anxiety has driven her to seek advice from a variety of sources. She may be trying to comply with instructions given by a variety of relatives, the Health Visitor, the general practitioner, good hearted neighbours and something she read in a book as well!

For example: Mrs A., aged 22

This patient was the younger of two children. Her mother was kindly but somewhat possessive and had some anxiety symptoms in adolescence. Her father was calm and placid but tended to let his wife take the initiative and make the decisions in the household. The patient was more close to her mother and this became even more marked when her elder brother died following a childhood infection. She had always been an anxious child and, because of her diffidence and her mother's understandable fears, had led a relatively sheltered life. She had met her husband at her local church and after a sedate courtship she duly married. Because of financial limitations the patient and her husband stayed on in her parents' home, using the top rooms of the house as a flat. The patient took considerable pride in running her flat and was quite an effective housewife. She continued a clerical job meanwhile. The sex relationship was unsatisfactory at first for both but gradually improved. The patient became pregnant six months after marriage. Early in pregnancy she complained of palpitations and dizzyness and consulted her general practitioner. Apart from a low blood pressure there were no abnormal findings and these symptoms were soon overlaid by morning sickness. At this point the patient gave up work. For a time she remained in bed and was nursed by her mother but by the fifth month was feeling much better and became active once more. She prepared the layette and other equipment and began to talk of the forthcoming baby with obvious pleasure. Towards the end of the pregnancy she again complained of palpitations, together with insomnia and indigestion. The birth was easy, but the patient had difficulty in adjusting to the hospital routine and pleaded to return home after the first few days. She showed considerable anxiety in handling her baby but began to breast-feed successfully. She was allowed home on the tenth day when her only complaint was some insomnia. Within a week, however, she again sought medical help with a multitude of symptoms, including a variety of aches and pains, palpitations, insomnia, tiredness and irritability. She complained that she had to give all her time to the baby, that he was restless and frequently cried, and she could not get off to sleep because she thought he was still crying and went again to see if all was well. A night sedative was prescribed and the patient reassured. The general practitioner heard nothing of the patient for a further month, when he was asked to visit by the husband. At this stage he found the patient in bed, complaining of all her previous symptoms. The baby was being cared for by her mother and the husband had been taking time off from work because he felt it unfair that his mother-in-law should look after the child as well as his wife, who felt unable to manage the housework and chores. Superficial questioning revealed that the patient had rapidly lost confidence in herself, in her relationship with the baby, and even her usual household duties. On the advice of a neighbour she had abandoned breast-feeding, but then found that she worried all day about the bottle and whether it was adequately sterilized, at the right temperature, and the right consistency. The husband said that she was in such a state when feeding the child that he had been relieved when her mother had taken over. At this point the patient felt so discouraged that she lacked the initiative even to take over the household cleaning and chores which had been neglected. She complained of severe insomnia with nightmares, fears that she would die, palpitations, and a number of other somatic symptoms.

Reactive depression

Some psychiatrists consider that there is no difference between reactive and endogenous depression, other than degree. It is true there may be difficulty in distinguishing between them in a borderline case and that in any one patient it may be possible to discover some elements which could be ascribed to either form of illness. Nevertheless in practice the majority of depressive illnesses can be sub-divided between the two types and certainly a different treatment and approach is indicated.

Many now consider that the 'four-day blues' is a short-lived reactive depression. It is much more commonly found in a patient delivered in hospital than in a patient delivered at home. It is often associated with a feeling of loneliness and frustration. Many patients freely express the need to return to familiar surroundings and to have their baby entirely to themselves.

Reactive depressions are common in the first few weeks after childbirth. The patient is under increased stress, often losing sleep, and with her pleasures and freedom limited, together with a real increase in her work load. A reactive depression is also likely to be precipitated by the loss of a child or a miscarriage, particularly late in pregnancy. Typically, the patient complains of feeling miserable and is tearful. She is aware of her symptoms, her sense of loss and the cause of it. Insomnia is common and, again, the patient has difficulty in getting off to sleep and her dreams are often clearly related to her practical problems, her lost child or other real source of stress. Any normal mother should experience some depression and sense of bereavement at the loss of a child. If, however, the mourning process becomes so marked or so prolonged that it interferes with her normal way of life and her ability to maintain her place in society, then one must assume there is a degree of illness present.

For example: Mrs B., aged 30 years

This patient was the eldest of three girls. There was no family history of any kind of psychiatric illness. Her mother had been somewhat hard and unaffectionate, while her father if anything too kindly, and had tended to 'spoil' her, giving her some preference over the other children. She had been over-attached to him and, although an attractive girl and courted by several men, did not marry until 28. She married a man ten years older than herself. She had little interest in children but, as her husband was anxious to have a family, had agreed to pregnancy early in marriage. The first child was born a year after marriage, but died in the first day of multiple congenital abnormalities. The patient was understandably depressed and tearful for several days but then appeared to accept the situation and, when she left hospital, was fairly cheerful. On her return home, however, to find evidence of the preparations she had made for the baby, she again became depressed, could not sleep, lost her interest in food, and continued to limit her life, rarely going out to meet friends or to any normal social gathering for several months. At this point her husband insisted on a further examination, largely because of her loss of weight. At this time she complained of depression. She said she still regretted having no child. She thought of the child constantly and had difficulty in getting off to sleep. She lost interest in food and also in any sexual relationship with her husband. She was frequently tearful and would weep at sentimental music. Further discussion revealed a number of other attitudes. There was considerable resentment at the fact that she had had all the trouble of pregnancy and labour 'for nothing' and some ill-concealed resentment towards her husband, who she knew wished her to go through the whole process again. This was a different attitude to that adopted towards her by her over-solicitous father. There was also considerable true regret at the loss of a child, but this regret was unduly prolonged because here again she had difficulty in accepting that she could have been disappointed in this way when most of her life her immediate wishes had been granted.

This case history demonstrates the common finding that any one symptom is the end result of a number of different mental mechanisms. This patient's depression was partly a normal grief reaction, it was also excessive in so far as her previous life had led her to expect that her wishes would be readily satisfied and it was also a way in which she could manipulate her husband and discourage him from persuading her to have another child.

It is easy to describe many of the neurotic reactions in the puerperium as depression, simply because many patients present with some tears whether of despair, frustration or true grief. It is preferable however to distinguish between the anxiety states showing emotional lability when tears are indeed frequent, reactive depression, when there is some true mourning process, and the more serious endogenous depression.

Hysteria

A diagnosis of hysteria has become much less common in recent years. It implies an emotional conflict which has been resolved unconsciously with the production of symptoms. Since the conflict has been resolved, the patient does not show anxiety or depression and, indeed, the classical emotional state is one of 'belle indifference'. The layman's picture of an 'hysterical woman' would be more correctly described as a woman showing emotionally uncontrolled behaviour, though some would refer to it as 'histrionics'. If we restrict hysteria to the above definition it is undoubtedly uncommon. Occasionally, it is associated with low intelligence and is said to be more common in primitive peoples. Gross hysterical symptoms, for example, blindness or paralysis, appearing soon after childbirth, suggest that the patient is completely unwilling to face the responsibility of her child. It should be remembered of course that the conflict lies between her instinctual desires which may well urge her towards a normal maternal attitude and some other part of her personality which rejects this. Occasionally, gross hysterical symptoms may appear in what is obvious to all as a simple flight from the situation, as when the girl with an illegitimate child abandons it and is found wandering in a 'fugue'. The chief hysterical symptoms are motor, that is paralyses, fits, and symptoms of this kind, sensory, with loss of sensation, and amnesic, as seen in the fugues and other conditions with loss of memory. Other conflicts may lead to the development of hysterical symptoms some weeks after childbirth, as in the following case.

Mrs D., aged 21 years

This patient had had a very formal upbringing in a strictly religious household. Her mother was a dullard, barely able to read or write and the patient herself had never reached the top standard of her elementary school. She had managed to hold down simple domestic work but one brief attempt to be a shop-assistant had failed because she could not manage the money. She was extremely shy and had few friends. To her surprise, she was courted by a somewhat uncouth youth who, because he was earning good money, pleased the patient's mother. The latter encouraged the engagement and the patient had very little say in the arrangements for her marriage. She was completely frigid and terrified to find herself pregnant after a few months' marriage. She failed to attend the antenatal clinic until a few weeks before the baby was due and had a difficult and prolonged labour in hospital. She was able to show the baby some limited affection but was unable to breast-feed and experienced some difficulty in managing the bottle feeds. Nevertheless, she returned home to her duties, but three weeks later suddenly complained of pains followed by weakness in the legs. She took to her bed and the husband summoned the doctor. Physical examination revealed that patient appeared to have rigidity of both lower limbs, some loss of sensation, but no true paralysis, and the reflexes could be obtained after diverting the patient's attention. Simple persuasion and encouragement produced no improvement in the symptoms. After some days she was transferred to hospital for further investigation. Here, too, no organic lesion was found and she was then referred to a psychiatrist. The patient denied all problems or stresses and insisted that, were she fit and well, she could return to her household duties. Fresh history-taking revealed that the symptoms began suddenly one night while in bed. The patient was so obviously hesitant in giving a further account that she was given some intravenous Pentothal until drowsiness supervened. In this state there was copious weeping and eventually she revealed that the symptoms commenced when her husband attempted intercourse and she, in terror of further pregnancy, shouted in pain and distress. Her husband desisted and the symptoms developed forthwith. The patient was not consciously aware of the true meaning of her symptoms. She had strong religious and moral convictions and she realized that to refuse her husband was against her principles which included those of being a dutiful wife. Nevertheless her experiences in pregnancy and childbirth had terrified her and, in the conflict between her duty and her fears, her symptoms provided the only satisfactory solution at the time. This patient rapidly improved and, following some discussion with her husband, adequate contraceptive techniques were accepted by both. Follow-up six months later showed the patient was still frigid but, although there had been no recurrence of her hysterical symptoms, she and her husband were barely on speaking terms and sexual relations had ceased. Her ability to care for her child was limited but the child, as is often the case even under adverse conditions, was thriving. Such a poor result was not surprising since only symptomatic treatment was given, and the patient had such very limited personality resources.

Obsessional states

Obsessional symptoms are of two main kinds, obsessional ruminations and obsessional compulsions. Sometimes they are mixed, the patient indulging in a number of compulsions in an attempt to control obsessional ruminations. Of all the neuroses, obsessional illness most commonly occurs with a family history.

Even when there is no frank family history of obsessional ill-ness, it will usually be found that one or other parent has clearly-marked obsessional traits in the personality. These personality traits, which include stubbornness, rigidity, excessive attention to detail, over-cleanliness and excessive concern for keeping rules, are frequently present in the patient before the illness appears. Another significant characteristic lies in the fact that, whereas most anxiety states tend to last for a few weeks with a tendency to spontaneous recovery, the duration of the obses-sional illness is more likely to be in months or even a year or two. Therefore an obsessional illness presenting in the puer-perium may well last until the child is a year or more old. Frequently the symptoms, although they appear the major problem to the patient, are of less significance to the family than the personality traits that go with them. When obessional symptoms develop for the first time in the months after child-birth in a patient who has not shown previous obsessional per-sonality traits or previous symptoms, it should be suspected that there is an underlying endogenous depressive illness. Many depressive illnesses have some obsessional symptoms together with other evidence of a gloomy concern with the ordinary details of everyday life. The obsessional symptoms occurring in a depressive illness carry the same prognosis as any other symptoms in the setting of depression.

The essential feature of obsessional ruminations is the recur-ring presence of unwelcome thoughts. Obviously, a thought which may be unwelcome for one person is not necessarily unwelcome for another. Frequently an unpleasant thought which comes to the patient's mind is associated with her baby. She may be aware of thoughts that the baby is abnormal or that the baby will die, or that she may harm it. A distinction should be made between such thoughts and impulses to harm the baby. Many women with thoughts of this kind are afraid that the thought will lead to the impulse which in turn will lead to the action. Obsessional compulsion may be based on an attempt to control such ruminations. For example, the patient may hide all sharp objects, lock up drawers where there are knives and hide her scissors, because of a persistent rumination that she may harm the baby on some sharp object. Sometimes, the ruminations may not be quite so clearly indicative of hostility to the child and may merely be that the child will injure itself or come to some harm against a sharp object, and this then justifies the compulsion which leads to all sharp objects being hidden. The person with obsessional traits who is preoccupied with cleanliness may find in the puerperium that the stress involved in keeping her infant clean leads to increasing tension and in turn increasing preoccupation with the baby's excretory functions. She may become fearful of contamination of other household objects with the baby's excreta or sometimes fear that some carelessness on her part will lead to contamination of the baby. Normal cleanliness and washing is replaced by repeated efforts which may lead to extravagant attempts to sterilize everything involved in baby care. The baby at this point may be in some danger from excessive attempts to keep its own person clean.

It is essential in the case of obsessional illness to remember that the symptom merely presents evidence of the conflicts and stress within the personality. Therapeutic preoccupation with the symptom and attempts to manipulate it or stop it may lead to the major problem lying in the patient's personality and the way she is managing her household to be neglected. It will usually be found that the patient with obsessional symptoms has already organized her household according to her own way of life and her own outlook and this, however compliant her relatives, may not be in the interest of their own health and emotional development. They may have accepted a routine and have become so used to it that they are reluctant to change. They may be afraid of alterations in the patient's attitudes towards them. Considerable support to all members of the family in their way of life and their adjustment to the patient's personality traits will always be found necessary in this kind of illness.

For example, Mrs W.

Her father had been a regular army officer and the patient clearly remembered her early life in which she travelled from one barracks to another, depending upon her father's postings. He was a very orderly and methodical man and her memories of her home and early years were entirely of his organization and insistence on cleanliness, punctuality, and orderliness. She and the other children were inspected each morning and again at night to see if their clothes were in good condition, appropriately stored and properly cared for. She remembered him coming into the house after his duty, when he would literally inspect the contents of his wife's kitchen, even looking under the mats to make sure there had been no dust improperly swept away. Her mother was a submissive woman who cheerfully accepted her husband's orders. The patient had conformed readily to her father's wishes and, being a bright intelligent child, had readily become his favourite. From an early age she had always kept herself clean and tidy and revelled in the praise she had received from her father as a result. Nevertheless, as she grew older her preoccupations with cleanliness began to cause difficulties. When her menstrual periods began she was considerably upset and for some months had a hand-washing compulsion. This was associated with some early sexual fantasies. Nevertheless, after some months, the hand-washing subsided and, as far as is known, she received no treatment or advice, nor at any time had she even consulted her parents. She had a number of short-lived love affairs in late adolescence but all came to nothing when the young men concerned began to make more amorous advances than she felt were acceptable in her conventional way of life. When she was 23 her younger sister married and this may well have led her to consider her next suitor more favourably. In any event, a year later she married a bank clerk who in some ways was almost as obsessional as herself. After some initial difficulties in sexual adjustment, she found herself rather more passionate than her husband and became pregnant within the first year. Like many obsessional patients, she insisted on conforming with every detail of the routine prescribed by her local antenatal clinic, religiously practising all her exercises, attending to her diet, and obeying every letter of the law as prescribed for her condition. The layette was complete and spotless and in every respect one could have assumed that this mother, of all those expecting their first child, was adequately prepared for all eventualities. In the maternity unit she was the model patient and had a relatively straight-forward labour. There was some difficulty on the maternity ward however as she asked specifically for guidance as to whether she should breast-feed or bottle-feed her infant. This particular unit made it clear that she should choose for herself which method she would prefer. The result of this advice was that she left the unit with the baby partially breast-fed, but supplemented with a bottle. At home she rapidly became preoccupied with the baby's bowel habits and asked for frequent reassurance from her relatives and the Health Visitor that the frequent motions in the baby's early days were normal. She began to feel that, having handled the nappy, her hands were in some way contaminated and she soon began excessive hand-washing. This became so severe and persistent that she had little time for other activities and began to neglect her other household chores. This then led to considerable secondary depression as she became aware of the dirt accumulating in other parts of the house. She enlisted the aid of her mother-in-law and asked for a Home Help through her local general practitioner. An assessment of the situation two months after her return home showed that much of her time was spent either in keeping her own person clean with hand-washing as a primary compulsion or, alternatively washing the baby, changing its nappy, and then indulging in an extensive ritual to ensure any dirt from the nappy could not possibly contaminate the rest of the household. The nappies were eventually boiled and if the least speck appeared on their surface boiled again. Since this was winter, her kitchen was constantly steamy and dripping with an endless array of nappies, on clothes-horses and lines from the ceiling. Much of this fruitless activity went on until late at night and she was getting up early in the morning, ostensibly because the baby woke then but also to return to her rituals. Interestingly enough, she did not complain of hand-washing herself but her husband realized at last that his wife's behaviour was outside the normal range. By this time he and the other relatives had learned to conform with his wife and they too were involved in some part of her rituals and played some part in their maintenance. He had to accept his share of the chores and the house-cleaning just as his mother did on her daily visits and as was expected of the Health Visitor also. The latter had realized the abnormality of the situation and had tried to explain the problem to the husband. The baby by this time was bottle-fed and had luckily adjusted fairly easily to a very rigid four-hourly routine. In the eventual development of the baby much depends on whether it has a nervous system which readily adapts to a rather rigid environment, which consists of regular feeds and, at an early age, strict toilet training. If this baby complied, as its mother had done in *her* early years, there would be no obvious problem which might lead to referral to a Child Guidance Clinic. If, on the other hand, this particular baby was unable to adjust to such a rigid environment, symptoms of one kind or another would be likely. The presence or absence of symptoms in the child does not necessarily give any clue to the degree of abnormality in the household.

CHAPTER SIX

The Psychoses (1)
The Organic Psychoses

As noted earlier the organic psychoses have become less common in most countries since the advent of effective antibiotics. The causes of the organic psychoses in pregnancy or the puerperium are exactly the same as those occurring at any other time. Some can be completely independent of childbearing; for example, a woman could be developing a cerebral tumour at the same time as she was pregnant. On the other hand, the majority of the toxic psychoses will be clearly related to the infections precipitated by the trauma of parturition.

During pregnancy, particularly in the later weeks, a severe toxaemia may well precipitate psychiatric symptoms. After the child's birth, infection is easily the commonest cause. Malaise, perhaps with loss of concentration or even mild confusion, is common enough but nowadays a full delirium is rare. Under present conditions a severe infection is usually necessary for this type of reaction. Severe anaemia also causes psychiatric symptoms. If it is of gradual onset it is more likely that the patient will complain simply of fatigue, lassitude, generalized depression and the clinical picture may resemble a neurosis. Anaemia of gradual onset may eventually lead to psychiatric symptoms but an acute one is more likely to do so.

For example, Mrs A.

Mrs A., a Nigerian woman, had come to this country a year previously. She had attended no antenatal clinic and was quite unknown to the hospital staff. Her child was born by Caesarian section at an unbooked confinement. There had been considerable blood loss. The day after operation she became very restless and excited, vividly hallucinated and resistant to attention.

She was transferred forthwith to a psychiatric hospital. On admission there she was found to be an obese patient with a very low blood pressure and at that time complaining of feeling very weak and lethargic. Blood tests showed a haemoglobin of 47 per cent but no evidence of any infection. Blood tests had also been taken at the maternity unit but the results had not been available at the time of the patient's transfer. Clinically it was noted that her hallucinations were largely visual and indeed these are more common in the organic states. There was prompt recovery with the appropriate treatment and within a few days the patient was symptom-free.

Drug-taking to excess has become more common in this country in recent years. Occasionally this can lead to a very puzzling clinical picture, unless the patient has admitted her habit to her physicians.

For example, Miss B.

Miss B. was an unmarried woman who came to the antenatal clinic a month before her child was due. Nothing abnormal was noted in antenatal examination and the child was born after a relatively brief labour. Two days after admission to the maternity unit however she became restless, tearful and somewhat excited. The next night she was unable to sleep and was found wandering up and down the ward floor. She screamed abuse at the night nurse. Sedation had very little effect and when examined in the early hours of the morning she was found to be restless, confused, disorientated, and visually hallucinated. A few hours later she had a succession of epileptic fits. She remained confused for some days and then gradually recovered. On recovery she admitted that she had been taking barbiturates in increasing dosage for some years, and in the weeks before her child was born had been taking up to thirty grains of sodium amytal daily. This medication ceased when she was admitted to hospital and her psychotic episode was entirely due to drug withdrawal.

Delirium is the chief psychosis associated with infections. It can occur following weeks of mild infection with a constant toxaemia when the patient has become gradually enfeebled. Alternatively, it may occur at the height of a severe acute infection. In general, delirium is a serious symptom and implies a severe toxic process. Although delirious symptoms appear readily in the very young and the very old, they are not common in middle life and are of more serious import in the healthy young woman than they would be in the enfeebled elderly. Initially the patient may complain of generalized aches and pains, fatigue and some confusion. It is notorious that delirious reactions tend to be worse at nights. Moreover, they commonly fluctuate so that an observer may find no evidence on one examination yet within the hour the patient may be floridly hallucinated.

The chief symptoms of delirium are an alteration in mood, an alteration in perception, and disturbance of memory and concentration. At first the patient feels anxious and apprehensive and may ask for reassurance from her attendants. Some patients complain of a feeling of impending catastrophe. Because of the feeling of fear, they may ask for relatives to be with them or for someone to hold their hand. They will be particularly fearful of being alone or being in the dark. Usually there is obvious heightening of fear as twilight approaches. At the height of the condition, the patient is obviously terrified and it is this feeling of fear, together with frightening hallucinatory experiences, which can lead to impulsive action. Changes in perception begin with illusions. Initially they may be similar to the experiences of children seeing faces in the fire but gradually the patient will see terrifying objects even on a blank wall and with minimal sensory stimuli to provoke them. Small stimuli may produce an exaggerated response, a small click sounds like a thunder-clap, an injection like being torn apart. Visual hallucinations are common in delirium but bizarre tactile experiences also occur. Patients may feel their skin is on fire or being burnt or having electric charges passed through it.

It is often noticeable that a patient can be distracted from delirious experiences by the presence of a friendly person or even by a stranger. For example, an examining doctor may look into the ward to see the patient lying staring at the ceiling, muttering, and apparently trying to evade hallucinated objects. He may go and speak to her and find his hand is taken and within a short time quite a coherent account of recent events may be obtained. If however he ceases to hold the patient's attention, she may rapidly fall back into a preoccupation with her previous hallucinations. It can usually be demonstrated that the patient has some confusion with memory disturbance, particularly of retention, and disorientation. Familiar objects and people are misidentified. An amnesia for the time of the delirium is common.

It is the combination of vivid hallucinations and feeling of terror which may lead the patient to precipitate action. She may attempt to leap out of the window or run out of the ward because of the terrifying objects which she feels will attack her. In few other conditions is good nursing care so essential. A skilled and tactful nurse can rapidly reduce the feeling of panic and by her careful and persistent attention draw the patient's attention away from her bizarre experiences and back to a normal conversation. It is usually essential to see that a nurse remains constantly with the patient while a delirium persists. It is not sufficient merely to keep a patient under observation in a single room which is visited at intervals. As with patients who are potentially suicidal, it is better to nurse her in a ward with other patients. A delirium is one of the few conditions where it is essential to wean the child. Obviously if the mother is toxic there is some risk to the infant of transfer of infection, quite apart from any harm which may come from the mother's restlessness or impulsive behaviour.

It is essential to treat the primary cause in any delirium with effective anti-biotics or other appropriate measures. On the other hand tranquillizers are equally essential and of these chlor-promazine is often the most effective. It is essential to give sufficient. The dosage should be rapidly doubled and redoubled, commencing with mg. 100 three times daily until an effective dosage is reached. As in other toxic conditions there may be an increased need for vitamins and it may be wise to give these parenterally.

CHAPTER SEVEN

The Psychoses (2)
Functional Psychoses: Schizophrenia

This illness is in many ways the most interesting, but also in many ways the most difficult to understand. Moreover, the literature gives very differing accounts as to its significance. As remarked upon in the introduction, Hemphill described a series with almost one hundred per cent failing to respond to treatment, whereas Martin's patients all improved. There is a further difficulty in that definitions of the illness vary—in some instances quite markedly—for example, some psychiatrists consider that a firm diagnosis can only be made if the disease shows an obvious tendency to deterioration. Others, including the author, consider that the disease has a very wide variety of manifestations, including brief episodes with a very good prognosis. It will be found that those psychiatrists, who believe that true schizophrenia from their point of view always carries a bad prognosis will describe those forms of the illness with a rapid recovery as 'schizophreniform episodes', or other convenient title. It is probable that with the advent of more effective methods of treatment the number of patients showing steady deterioration is rapidly becoming less and the majority of psychiatrists are now willing to make a diagnosis of schizophrenia, even when the patient makes a good recovery.

Most studies show that there will be a clear family history of schizophrenia in one or other parent in about fifteen per cent of cases. A larger percentage will give a history of psychosis in more distant relatives and also of abnormal personalities, alcoholism or other psychiatric disorder more frequently than would be expected in an ordinary family tree. The family history should be taken more seriously if there is a history of schizophrenia in the mother or sisters, particularly if the illness developed following childbirth. It is surprising to find that although the mother and perhaps grandmother had schizophrenic illnesses following childbirth, the prognosis is not necessarily a bad one, should their child develop the same illness in her turn. Apart from any history indicating an obvious breakdown, care should be taken to determine the precise meaning of changes in personality in the patient's mother following childbirth. Schizophrenia may develop without florid symptoms, but lead to insidious personality changes. This may be remembered clearly by the patient or other relatives though its true significance may have escaped them and also the mother's medical attendants. For example, one patient was seen showing severe insomnia, agitation, and some bizarre symptoms with anxiety eleven days after the birth of her child. Her mother had never had a known psychiatric illness, but the patient remembered that, after the birth of her last child, she had become very faddy with her food and lived for many years on a severely restricted diet, which she insisted on eating by herself, so that the family was brought up to remember their mother running the household and preparing their meals while disappearing to eat her own in seclusion. The mother had also shown other evidence of personality change with loss of feeling towards her children and a tendency to retire from any normal social life. At no time, however, had she sought medical assistance and the changes had developed so insidiously that they had been accepted as within normal limits.

It used to be a traditional belief that schizophrenia developed in patients who showed obvious 'schizoid' personality traits; that is they were retiring, introverted, awkward with strangers, often over-sensitive, and tending to day-dream. It was suggested that this type of personality, together with the asthenic body build predisposed to the development of schizophrenia. More recent studies, however, have shown that the illness may occur in a wide variety of personality types and in many there appears to have been no forewarning in the patient's previous personality or reaction to stress. It is possible that the idea that

schizophrenia developed only in people with limited personalities came as a result of studies on those patients who were
eventually treated for long periods in mental hospitals. For
obvious reasons it is likely that those patients with limited
personalities would be those with the least ability to recover
from the illness and therefore the more likely to form the core
of any long-term mental hospital population.

Some recent work has suggested that the family environment
in early life can predispose the patient towards a schizophrenic
illness. In particular, the 'schizophrenogenic' mother has been
described who sets double standards for her children and makes
any consistent relationship to reality difficult for them. Many of
the published case histories, however, suggest that simple
inheritance could as easily explain the findings as the assumption that method of the upbringing played the major part.
Certainly many patients with schizophrenia seem to have had
a very understanding upbringing, nor does schizophrenia seem
more common in the child from a broken home or with a clear
history of deliberate ill-treatment. As would be expected,
however, patients with personality limitations will find it more
difficult to overcome the handicaps imposed by an illness like
schizophrenia.

It will usually be found that a schizophrenic illness follows an
emotional stress but quite often there is some delay of days—or
even weeks—before the symptoms appear. Frequently relatives
will state that between the stress and the onset of symptoms, the
patient seemed bewildered or in some way unable to react with
normal emotional expression. It is difficult to decide whether
this is merely a latent period or the first symptoms of the illness.
It is certainly a common observation that florid symptoms very
rarely develop during childbirth itself, but tend to appear a few
days later or insidiously—even months later. There is no
evidence that physical trauma, infection, or similar stress is more
common in the patient who develops schizophrenia than the
rest of the population. On the other hand emotional stress, in particular insecurity and uncertainty do seem to be common factors.

The classical symptoms of schizophrenia are due to changes in thinking and changes in emotional reactions. The changes in thinking lead the patient to complain of difficulty in concentration and feelings of confusion. There is often difficulty in making decisions and the patient may ask the same question on numerous occasions. A particular form of thought disorder will often develop. In this the patient often finds her train of thought interrupted so that she cannot maintain a consistent line of thinking and also, perhaps the reverse of this loss of her train of thought, that irrelevant words, phrases, or ideas come to mind when she does not want them. In the retarded patient this may be a very slow process but in the excited patient there may be a terrifying awareness of the ideas crowding into the head which cannot be controlled. As a result of thought disorder, the patient's conversation tends to become restricted with a tendency to keep strictly to concrete and literal interpretations. With more severe disorder still, sentences become replaced by disjointed phrases and eventually a meaningless babble of words—'word salad'. Patients with schizophrenia may attempt to explain themselves in a bizarre fashion, or by using new words—'neologisms'—which have special meaning for the patient but are incomprehensible to others. Patients may attempt to explain their disordered thinking processes and ascribe an intrusion of thoughts to the action of machines or radio waves. Such explanations are of course delusions and, as a rule, delusions should be considered late symptoms and the diagnosis made before these have developed. In the early stages, the patient may be aware of thoughts appearing in her head and may accept these as being her own production, even if unusual. There is no clear borderline between this kind of experience and similar thoughts appearing to come from outside the patient as hallucinatory voices. Frequently schizophrenic hallucinations appear meaningless and pointless but, in the acute stage of the illness, they may be of serious import if, for example, they urge the patient to impulsive action.

The emotional changes are an essential part of the schizophrenic illness. They consist of loss of emotional reaction
('flattening') and inappropriate (incongruous) emotions. Initially, the patient may complain that she feels different in some
way. It is characteristic that the patient finds it very difficult to
put this into words or to have the feeling that others understand
her. She may complain of feeling unreal or dreamy. Quite
commonly, she also feels bewildered with an undercurrent of
fear. She may feel that the world is changing around her and
potentially threatening her. It is in these early stages that many
patients cling to those around them, ask for help and, as noted
earlier, make repeated requests over trifling issues. This is often
referred to as 'reality testing' and does imply that the patient is
trying to distinguish between her normal world and relationships and those which are now appearing as a result of the
illness. The patient's attitude towards those around her may
change dramatically once the initial phase of anxiety and
perplexity is passed. She may then feel that those around her
undoubtedly intend harm and she may accuse her husband of
neglecting her, ill-treating her, or consorting with other
women. She may feel that the nursing staff are hostile to her and
intend to do her or the baby some harm. It is usually obvious
that the patient's delusions stem from the change in feeling and
thinking and that attempts to explain or correct these delusions
are fruitless, since the convictions are rooted in the patient's
altered feelings.

Many patients with schizophrenia, particularly in the early
stages, complain of depressive symptoms. There may be true
unhappiness and this is often related to the patient's awareness
of her condition. Some patients sense that their personality is
disintegrating and are terrified of this experience. Many other
patients, however, complain of depression, but enquiry will
show this does not mean unhappiness or misery, as ordinarily
understood, but is their attempt to explain what is happening.
A patient who complains of depression should always be asked
exactly what it means to her and, if the answer is confusion,

bewilderment, and the loss of concentration, or similar statements, suspicion should be aroused that the patient does not have a simple depressive illness. Many patients with an obvious schizophrenic illness have had an initial diagnosis of depressive reaction and ineffectual treatment instituted.

It is not surprising that with the difficulty in thinking and the changes in the emotional state, the patient's ability to interact with her environment should be seriously handicapped. Those around her will sense that she is a different sort of person, and quite often the relatives will find it very difficult to explain the precise difficulties this causes. Personality change, however, is one of the most consistent signs noted by those who have previously known the patient. Her ability to manage and organize her household will be severely handicapped by thought disorder, and the most tolerant husband will feel frustrated when his normal affectionate approaches are rebuffed and he feels that his wife is in some way a different person. As noted earlier, it is important to treat the patient before the development of florid hallucinations and delusions make the diagnosis obvious to all. Relatives can be quite remarkably tolerant as well as intolerant of schizophrenic illness. For example, one husband admitted that his wife had been hallucinated for two years but said he had not worried about it until she had a baby and then he realized it might have some effect on the baby's upbringing! One of the commonest fears is that the patient with schizophrenia will harm her baby, perhaps in some bizarre or terrible way. In practice, however, it is very rare to find that a patient with schizophrenia does actively attack her child or involve the child in a dangerous situation as a result of delusions. Much the greater risk is that the child will be neglected and the patient who is bewildered by thought disorder and preoccupied with the bizarre changes in herself may be oblivious to her child's crying and discomfort. This is by no means a general rule, however, since many mothers—even with a florid schizophrenic illness and considerable disturbance of behaviour—may show warmth of affect to their baby and give good standards of care even when all other emotional relationships are disrupted.

Many schizophrenic patients not only feel that the world around them is changing but also feel that their own body has changed in some peculiar fashion. Some merely state that their body feels different or has changed. They may be found looking into a mirror to see if there is anything visible. Others will locate this change and may describe it in bizarre terms. They may say that they feel that their head has only one side to it, or their heart has moved to the other side of their body, or that strange electrical charges run up and down inside them. Delusions with a sexual content are common. Some patients say they feel they are changing into a man or may insist that this change has already occurred. Others insist some peculiar sexual activity is being forced upon them, perhaps at night when they are asleep. They may accuse anyone around them of being implicated. Beliefs that their body has changed, smells peculiarly or is abnormal or grotesque in some form or another will occasionally be a presenting symptom and take the patient to her general practitioner. The patient may insist on further investigation, perhaps believing that she smells offensively when, in fact, she is a very fastidious person. This type of insistence on investigation of a non-existent symptom should alert the practitioner to assess the patient's mental state further.

Delusional ideas may centre around the baby. Some women will insist the baby is dead or that it is deformed. Delusions of this kind have been used to support the theory that hostility to the baby was the universal cause of psychiatric breakdown in the puerperium and in the case of schizophrenia hostility showed itself in this kind of delusion. Other mothers however will insist they have a beautiful baby when they have a deformed one or, alternatively, they have twins when they have only one child. This makes it very difficult to accept that any one type of psychodynamics can be accepted in this condition. The emotional incongruity previously described may be very apparent indeed when major psychotic symptoms are centred on the child. It is quite bewildering to the observer to hear a woman deny her baby exists yet fondle it and breast-feed it. Similarly, she may state categorically that the baby is dead, yet treat it perfectly well and with a good show of affection. Mothers with a schizophrenic excitement who show very considerable disturbance of behaviour towards those around them may nevertheless become calm and relaxed while breast-feeding their child and this can occur when all other reactions are incongruous, whereas the relationship with the baby may be the only normal one left. It is because of these clinical observations, apart from the known therapeutic results, that make it preferable to treat mother and baby together even when the mother has such a major functional psychosis as schizophrenia.

When mother and baby are kept together, when the former has a schizophrenic illness, there are some real risks which must be remembered. Although the risk of deliberate injury to the child is almost non-existent, the risk of neglect is real. It is often easy to observe that a schizophrenic mother fails to respond to her child's demands. She may pick the child up and observe it closely while the child wails in obvious hunger or distress. Although the patient is obviously aware of the situation, she may take no steps either to comfort the child, cuddle it, provide it with food, or in any other way attempt to relieve its distress. Some patients are aware of this and complain that they lack feeling for their child and seem quite unable to respond to its demands. This loss of feeling can of course occur in other conditions too but may be one of the chief problems in the management of the mother and child in this particular condition. Fortunately, with effective treatment, good affect for the baby can return, even in the patient who appears initially to be completely lacking in any normal maternal feelings. The prognosis will of course be very much better if it is known that the patient normally has good affective responses to those around her and better still if it is known that she has at

some time had good affect either for this child or another.
A schizophrenic illness or episode is a serious matter and even
if the acute symptoms only last for a few days, it is probably
wise to assume that the patient should remain under some degree
of medical observation for at least the next year. This observation can be discreet through occasional visits on the part of the
general practitioner, by adequate discussion with the husband
or—and sometimes this may be the best of all—through routine
visits by the Health Visitor. It should be remembered that it is
not only the florid, acute disturbance that schizophrenia
occasionally produces which is of serious import, but also the
insidious personality change, which can be a disaster in the
household. In general, the acute episodes are readily recognized
and, if treated early, the results of treatment are good. Insidious
personality change is often missed, treatment is instituted late
and, in this situation, the prognosis is much less satisfactory.

Husbands frequently ask how they should attempt to make a
relationship with their wives again once she has had a schizophrenic illness. Much will depend on the husband's own
emotional state and maturity and his ability to give spontaneous
affection. Many patients with schizophrenia lack initiative and
also lack the emotional warmth to initiate human relationships.
If the husband can take the initiative, can make the effort to
make conversation with his wife, to initiate social activities, to
stimulate her to household organization, all these will help the
patient to regain a routine which will keep her in touch with
reality and the satisfactions of everyday life. Sexual relations,
similarly, are not only a practical matter but mean a considerable degree of emotional interaction. Many patients with
schizophrenia find sex relationships one of the more satisfactory
ways in which they can make and develop a human relationship
again. It is essential that both patient and her husband should
know of the risk of relapse should there be any further pregnancy. The patient who has had a serious schizophrenic illness
and already has two or three children should be advised to
have no more, and seriously consider a sterilization.

Another situation in which schizophrenia may well carry a poor prognosis is when a patient has an illegitimate child and a puerperal schizophrenic illness. This particular combination carries a very poor prognosis indeed. Although the initial breakdown will respond to treatment as well as in other situations, it is inevitable that the young mother will have very considerable stresses over the years if she has no husband to support her. If the girl's parents are willing to support her and stand by her, obviously the situation is more hopeful. However, it must be remembered that her parents not only have the difficulty of accepting a daughter with an illegitimate child, but also a daughter who has had a mental illness who will require more support, more understanding and more care than she had previously. It is understandable that they may well be more likely to reject her or, alternatively, be more intolerant than parents who have a daughter with only one of these handicaps. It is the author's experience that it is highly unlikely that a girl who has an illegitimate child and a schizophrenic illness will bring the child up. Many will attempt to do so because, as previously noted, the emotional tie between mother and baby may be very strong, even when the mother has schizophrenia. Nevertheless, relapse under the stress of trying to care for the child and support herself is much more common in this situation. Some mothers, however, try to readjust to ordinary life, relapse, have further treatment, return once more, and throughout try to keep their child. Only after two or three years' repeated relapses, it may become apparent to all that there is no possible future in the relationship. For this reason, very serious thought should be given very early in the illness, whether in this particular situation there is any point in trying to maintain the mother/baby relationship. Usually, it is kinder and less traumatic for the patient to be separated from the baby at the onset of the illness. It is for this reason that an accurate diagnosis is essential, since the risks are not so great in other psychiatric conditions with illegitimacy. If the patient with schizophrenia and an illegitimate child is admitted to hospital and treated effectively without the baby, it may be easier for her to accept the bereavement and make a fresh start as a single girl without the additional problems and responsibilities of a child. To admit them both to a Mother and Baby Unit and then treat the mother, only when her time comes to leave hospital to separate her from the child, is not only cruel but for obvious reasons must increase the risk of relapse, rather than reduce it. From the author's unit for the mothers with schizophrenia there has only been one patient with an illegitimate child who, over the years, was able to keep the child with her and maintain a normal life and, in this case, the patient married within a few months of leaving hospital and thus provided herself with the essential support she needed. A similar situation holds when the husband deserts his wife. Unless she has some other relative who gives her a very considerable degree of emotional and financial support, it is unlikely in the long run that she will be able to maintain herself and the child in a stable relationship. Attempts to reunite a husband and wife, when the wife has schizophrenia, as a rule are doomed to failure. The husband, who has already deserted his wife because of this illness, is unlikely to have the emotional warmth or sympathy for her condition which are absolutely essential and need to be maintained not only for short periods, but frequently for many years if the marriage is to continue.

Case histories

The clinical picture in schizophrenia can vary more than in any other condition. For this reason some brief illustrative case histories will be given. The first is that of the typical acute schizophrenic illness, developing in the first week of the puerperium.

Mrs N.

This attractive and intelligent young woman was married to a professional man. Two years after marriage she became pregnant with a planned baby. They moved into a convenient apartment shortly before the baby was due. She remained well throughout the pregnancy apart from some morning sickness for which she required no treatment. The baby was delivered in a private maternity home by the obstetrician of her choice. Labour lasted for twenty-four hours and there was eventually a spontaneous delivery with a small tear. Her physical condition was good however and she seemed alert and cheerful when her husband visited later the same day. It was noted however that she failed to sleep for the first two nights after childbirth and had only fitful sleep with sedation on the third night. The following day she was weeping and irritable and began to complain of conditions in the nursing home. She seemed reassured by her husband's visit but again obtained little sleep. The next day when the husband visited, she not only complained of conditions, as previously, but also alleged that because of her complaints she was being victimized. The husband had an interview with the ward sister but tended to side with his wife. The next day while at work he received an urgent summons asking him to visit his wife. On his arrival, he found his wife in her room weeping. She shouted at the nurse in attendance and insisted that she should be taken home forthwith. She gave a detailed account of various annoyances and slights which she felt the nurses had put upon her. The husband was enraged at this, also accused the nurses of neglecting his wife, ordered a taxi and took her home. He arranged for a relative to stay with his wife and asked his general practitioner to take over her care. His wife seemed much calmer in her own home but again failed to sleep that night. She woke her husband in the small hours and gave him a somewhat disjointed and graphic account of her experiences in labour. She became increasingly excited. The husband eventually became alarmed and said that he would send for the doctor. At this point his wife leapt out of bed and ran screaming out of the flat in her night-clothes. She was eventually stopped by a passing policeman and with great difficulty returned to the flat. When seen in consultation the next day, she was dishevelled, restless, and voluble. It was difficult to follow the trend of her conversation. At intervals she accused the staff of the maternity unit of having injured her in some way and also of having made the baby deformed, though the baby was quite normal. When questions were asked, she listened but frequently answered quite irrelevantly while on other occasions not at all. Her behaviour suggested she was hallucinated. She was admitted to a psychiatric unit and treated with chlorpromazine. She had a good night's sleep following chlorpromazine mg 200 t.d.s. together with six grains of sodium amytal at night. The next day she was able to give a more coherent history, confirmed that she was hallucinated and could still hear the voices of the ward sisters making offensive and insulting remarks about her. She still believed her baby to be deformed though she could point to no abnormality when given the opportunity. In spite of her statements she was able to give the baby obvious affection and was breast-feeding successfully.

A review of the history showed that she was an only child. Her mother had had a long period of ill-health following the patient's birth and had been advised to have no more children. The husband described his mother-in-law as being a vague impractical sort of person who had showed singularly little feeling either to her husband or child, though able to run a fairly simple household competently. Unfortunately, the patient's father was dead and no more accurate account of his wife's breakdown was ever obtained. The patient herself had normal milestones, with no particular neurotic traits and, although somewhat over-indulged as a child by her father, had showed none of the so-called schizoid traits prior to her illness. She had been a good scholar and trained as a physiotherapist prior to her marriage.

This case history demonstrates the relatively acute onset in the early days of the puerperium in a woman with no previous history, nor any clue to suggest that breakdown was possible other than the suspicious family history.

Mrs B.

This patient was from a working-class family with no family history of mental illness of any kind. Although poor, she was well-treated as a child and had considerable affection from both parents. She was regarded as somewhat sensitive and shy but not more so than many other girls. She was an average scholar and became a shop-assistant before her marriage. She married at the age of twenty. Her husband was five years the senior and worked as a clerk in the Inland Revenue. He was a pleasant but somewhat inadequate man with very few interests or hobbies. His wife said he came home in the evening, read his paper, and went to bed and had no secret vices nor particular virtues either. He was content to leave the running of the house to his wife and she made most of the decisions up to the time of their first child. The first child was born a year after marriage. Its birth was not entirely welcome as they had to leave furnished rooms to move to a less convenient flat, where the baby was accepted. The child was born in hospital and there were no physical complications. On return home, the husband noticed no particular change in his wife at the time. She however complained of increasing tiredness and difficulty in managing the household. She dropped her social activities completely and ceased to meet her friends. Her husband ascribed this to the results of childbirth and merely thought it took his wife a long time to recover. She never did return to her previous level of activity or competence and became pregnant again two years after the first child. At the beginning of her pregnancy she experienced considerable anxiety, being worried that she would be quite unable to manage another infant. During the middle months of pregnancy however she felt very well and her old competence reasserted itself. She reorganized her household and tidied up the flat in preparation for the new baby.

The second child too was born in hospital without any unusual circumstances. She returned home having complained of no difficulties or symptoms. Her husband however found that meals were rarely prepared for him when he came home at night and he, in turn, began to have a meal on the way back from his work so that he had no difficulty on this score. He noticed that the house became increasingly untidy and dirty and that the baby's crying was often ignored. His wife failed to attend the post-natal clinic and, after the first two visits, refused to allow the Health Visitor in to see the child. The patient breast-fed the child successfully and, in spite of a steady deterioration in her ability to run the home and her general standards of care in the household, there were no unusual incidents until the baby was seven months. At this age, the child developed a chest infection, possibly associated with erupting teeth. The mother ignored this but did complain to her husband that the child had gone off its food. He told her she should take it to the doctor but, when he found she had not done so the next day, he called the general practitioner in. By this time the child had quite severe broncho-pneumonia and had to be admitted to a paediatric unit where it made a good recovery. On the baby's return home however it developed a fresh infection a week later and was again seriously ill and re-quired re-admission. At this point, the general practitioner noticed that the mother's reaction to these events seemed very shallow and she showed a singular lack of concern. When the doctor mentioned this to the patient's husband, he confirmed that she had become quite a different person from the girl he had married.

On examination at this time, the patient looked untidy and unwashed. She was able to give quite a clear account of herself and recent events, though she complained of some difficulty in concentration and an inability to plan the day. She showed very considerable flattening of affect. She showed no concern for her child who had been desperately ill twice within recent weeks and was at that time in hospital. She had not troubled to visit nor expressed any concern in the child's progress. She was aware of the squalor of her home, the lack of cleanliness and the evidence of disorder but, although she said that the house needed a good spring-clean, she said this with a shallow smile and showed no impulse or initiative to carry out this task. During the interview it was noticeable that at times her attention wandered and she seemed to be preoccupied with her own thoughts. Further enquiry revealed that she had a variety of bizarre ideas coming into her head and at times was hallucinated. She said that she had had similar feelings after the first child but that these had gradually subsided, though she had not felt really well until the middle of the second pregnancy.

This case history illustrates the development of an insidious schizophrenic illness with flattening of affect as the most prominent symptom. She also had a mild degree of thought disorder, sufficient to disorganize her planning and initiative. This, together with the lack of drive, led to the social and personality deterioration so obvious to the outsider but to which the husband had gradually become accustomed.

A third case history will illustrate yet another facet of this remarkable disease.

Mrs C.

This patient also gave no history of any family mental illness nor any neurotic or personality defects in her own early life. She married at eighteen and had her first child at the age of twenty-one. Her marriage seemed happy and with no unusual stresses. About a fortnight after the birth of the child, her husband noticed on his return home from work that she was unusually quiet and when he spoke to her she became tearful. She could give no explanation for this and he assumed that it was merely a reaction to the child's birth. She failed to improve however and became more withdrawn, less ready to talk and less able to manage day-to-day affairs. The weeping gradually stopped and for a time her husband thought she had improved. When the baby was a month old he returned home one evening to find his wife had returned to her bed soon after he left the house and had failed to feed the child all day. As she had been breast-feeding and he found the baby crying, he placed the child to the breast where it obtained an adequate meal, though its mother took no notice and stared at the ceiling throughout the whole proceedings. Her husband was only able to obtain an occasional 'yes' or 'no' to his questions. He sent for his general practitioner forthwith. When this patient was examined the next day, she was in stupor. She made no response to questioning though was obviously conscious and awake. She showed a limited response to painful stimuli but would make no reply to questions nor comply with simple commands. When attempts were made to move her, she resisted. She also resisted efforts to offer her food or drink. Her husband said she had been incontinent during the night. In spite of this, he had again placed the baby to the breast in the morning and the baby once more had taken an adequate feed and was sleeping peacefully at the time of the visit.

This case history illustrates the development of schizophrenic stupor and the history, as given by the husband and later confirmed by his wife, showed that there had initially been a phase of depression but after a few days this had passed and the patient had become more negativistic, and withdrawn as the schizophrenic illness had become more apparent. It should also be noted that in spite of the severity of her mental illness there was no interference with lactation.

CHAPTER EIGHT

The Psychoses (2)
Functional Psychoses: Manic Depressive Illness

This type of illness is the most common of the functional psychoses. Two-thirds of all cases can be expected to give a positive family history. Although depressive episodes are much the more common, any patient who has had a depressive episode also carries the risk of a manic attack at some time in her life. Some patients have a regular cycle in which a brief manic episode, perhaps lasting a few days, is then followed by a depressive attack lasting some months. It is to be remembered that any stress which may precipitate a depression may also precipitate mania. In general it is fair to say manic-depressive illnesses tend to develop towards middle life, and perhaps become increasingly common at the end of that part of life's span. For obvious reasons therefore such illnesses are uncommon in the young woman but tend to be more common as she nears middle-age. This is of some importance both in differential diagnosis and in prognosis. An episode of excitement in a young woman is unlikely to be mania and a diagnosis of schizophrenia or a toxic condition is more likely. A severe depressive illness occurring after a first child in a relatively young woman will probably not recur following a second child; the odds against this are about four to one. On the other hand, a similar depressive illness in a woman of forty carries a different prognosis. Should she have a further child a year or two later a further depression is much more likely than in the case of the younger woman. There are differences in prognosis and relapse rates in the available statistics, this being largely accounted for by variations in diagnostic criteria. In particular, there is likely to be a difference in the prognosis in those depressions of sufficient severity to compel the patient's admission to a mental hospital compared with those depressions which are still treatable on an out-patient or domiciliary basis.

Fortunately mania is rare in the puerperium. The practitioner will see at least a hundred depressions to every manic episode. In the author's experience, manic episodes tend to occur earlier in the weeks following childbirth than depressive illnesses. As noted earlier, acute excitements occurring in the first weeks after childbirth are much more likely to be schizophrenic in nature than manic. Nevertheless, the latter illness does occasionally occur.

For example, Mrs K.

She came from a professional family. Her mother had had a menopausal depression followed by several relapses in the following ten years, but in her old age had remained stable. The patient had had a happy home life, had been a good scholar and left school to go to teacher-training college. After two years as a teacher, she married and became pregnant almost at once. She had no difficulties during pregnancy and was described by her husband as being very fit and happy with normal preoccupations and expectations for child-rearing. She had her child in hospital and returned home a week later. During the second week of her return home she began to experience difficulty in sleeping, this characteristically developed as early waking. The first night or two this was attributed to her concern over the baby's feed, but in the succeeding nights she began to wake earlier and earlier. She began to get up and, her husband noted, seemed to be unduly active and to have an excess of energy. She began to clean and tidy the house in the small hours and on one occasion he woke at four a.m. to hear his wife singing whilst cleaning out the bathroom. This excess of energy however did not mean that the household was run the more efficiently. On return from work the husband found some chores were incomplete while other quite unnecessary work had been done. His wife was full of plans but these changed so rapidly that none initiated were satisfactorily completed. She insisted that she

was quite well but the husband noted that the baby was beginning to suffer. She would pick the child up, begin to breast-
feed but, before the child could complete the feed, it was
placed down again and its wails ignored or explained away far
too light-heartedly. It was the baby's evident distress which led
the husband to ask for help from the Health Visitor and she,
in turn, reported the problem to the general practitioner. When
the doctor arrived at the house, the patient met him at the door,
partially clad, but nevertheless flung the door open to the full
view of passers-by. She proudly showed him round the house,
the new baby, the cot, and the preparations for the future.
She maintained a constant pressure of talk, interspersed with
occasional wisecracks and comic remarks mostly in keeping but
some of them rather crude. Her general behaviour was noisy
and boisterous and quite different from her usual composed and
competent self. She was very distractable and acted on the
impulse of the moment. She caused her husband considerable
embarrassment by suddenly deciding to disrobe completely in
the middle of the living-room so that the doctor could complete
his examination. Physically, she was fit but of the pyknic build
which is commonly found in this type of illness. The distracta-
bility shown by this patient, so that her conversation could be
turned readily from one subject to another, and any chance
move or gesture was likely to bring some response, was typical
of the manic state and contrasted with the schizophrenic patient
who would have been preoccupied and absorbed with her inner
experiences and fantasies.

The endogenous depressions include some of the most
serious illnesses carrying the gravest risk to the life of both
mother and child. It should be made clear that infanticide and
suicide are rarities but nevertheless one such incident in a
practice will carry emotional overtones in the neighbourhood
for many years to come. Knowledge of these disasters is universal. Unfortunately, each fresh occurrence is liable to bring
with it newspaper headlines and much comment and discussion.
It is inevitable that women, when they are depressed, and have

morbid thoughts are likely to consider these possibilities and both the patient and her relatives may give far too great a weight to these risks. It is not uncommon to find that a mother and her baby have been parted at the first hint of depression because of the fear that harm will come. The very fact of separation may merely reinforce the woman's guilt feelings and also tell her that her self-control is no longer trusted by those around her. This in turn may merely make the risk of some harm the greater rather than lessening the danger. Nevertheless it must be admitted that the real risk of injury to the child lies in the severe depressive illness far more than any other psychiatric state. Moreover, the bulk of women who consider infanticide are suicidal risks too.

Some endogeneous depressive illnesses begin early in the puerperium, others two to four months after the child is born. As a rule, the onset is insidious and at first ordinary fatigue and worry is accepted as a natural explanation of the situation. It is particularly important to remember that severe depressions may occur in a woman of previous good personality, sociable, hard-working and competent, in fact the very person of whom her neighbours say: 'I would never imagine she could have a nervous breakdown.' A second factor which can be deceiving is the patient's tendency to self-reproach. A patient with this type of depression will tend to blame herself. She may accept the advice of others to 'pull her socks up' or to 'try harder' and may feel that the difficulties she is experiencing are entirely her own fault. If she believes the fault is entirely her own, it then becomes understandable that she should not seek medical help or trouble to bother others with her difficulties. Many of the traditional depressive symptoms will be present in these patients. Self-reproach has already been mentioned. Retardation is common, many somatic symptoms, including constipation, indigestion, and general sluggishness are evident. In many depressions symptoms are worse in the early part of the day and there is improvement as the day wears on. This particular symptom is obscured in the puerperal depression because of the presence of the baby. A mother who is regularly wakened in the early hours of the morning may have great difficulty in distinguishing between this and the early waking of a depression. Similarly the demands of the child may make it difficult for her to distinguish whether her mood is indeed better in the morning or the evening.

Patients with depression often show a characteristic change towards their child. Initially, there is often evidence of oversolicitousness and an attempt to improve standards of care. Together with this can often be noticed some irritability though the patient will often express some guilt that she should feel this. Often the patient will feel that her baby is in some way ill or abnormal and this may be the first sign that brings the patient to the family doctor's notice. She may think the child is unusually backward or some small birthmark carries an ominous implication. Trivial symptoms may be interpreted as evidence of serious disease. The minor abnormalities or asymmetry so commonly noted in a baby, lead to endless preoccupation and rumination as to their possible cause. It is too easy to reassure these patients that nothing is wrong with their child. It is essential to recognize the difference between this type of patient and the one who is merely anxious. In the anxious patient some measure of reassurance is indeed sought by the patient and, if accompanied by discussion of her other difficulties, may help her. In the case of the depressive however she is not seeking reassurance but merely telling the world and her doctor in particular that her feelings towards the baby have changed and are no longer within the range of normal maternal anxiety.

For example, Mrs P., aged 35

This patient had been a hard-working woman who had nursed her mother through considerable chronic ill-health until she died when the patient was thirty. It was only at this age that the patient allowed herself to consider the possibility of marriage. Even so, she did not marry until thirty-three and at that point married a rather dour, humourless man who, although a good provider from the material point of view, showed relatively little affection towards the patient. She had considerable sickness during pregnancy and a difficult labour. Breast-feeding was never established satisfactorily and she returned home with the baby already on the bottle. At home, she managed well for the first two months, giving the baby a good standard of care, and appearing to return to her previous level of health. She showed considerable pride in her child and joined in with the local group of young mothers in attendances at the post-natal clinic and infant welfare meetings. At about this time, she mentioned to the Health Visitor that she thought her child's head was an unusual shape. She was reassured and no further comment arose until a week later when she made the same comment to the doctor in the welfare clinic. She told the doctor that she had seen another child who was a Mongol and thought that her own child had a similar shaped head. She was again reassured and, although her own baby's head was undoubtedly round, the difference between this and the typical Mongol and the absence of the other features of Mongolism were explained to her. Before the next baby clinic the general practitioner was called to see her after she had taken an overdose at home.

A full reconstruction of the history showed that she had been depressed for two or three weeks. Her husband had not noticed this but her next-door neighbour had become aware that the patient had tended to stay indoors instead of going out and seemed unable to get through her ordinary daily chores. The Health Visitor confirmed that she had seemed quieter and more subdued and the patient herself confirmed that she had felt depressed. At times she thought she had married far too late in life, and that she had not tried hard enough, and would never make a success of her marriage. It was in this setting that she began to feel that something was wrong with the child. The most ominous symptom which was not revealed until after the incident with the overdose, was the patient's admission that she felt she could not trust herself with the baby in the early part of the day when it cried and she had for the last week made a practice of placing the child outside the house in its pram while she stayed indoors to do the chores. A careful review of her feelings at the time showed that she was fearful that the child's crying would make her so irritated that she would attack it.

This patient made a full recovery with treatment but in her illness can be seen all the symptoms which can, in the occasional case, lead to tragedy: self-reproach, delusional ideas (to believe one's child a Mongol when there is no evidence of this is a delusion), mounting hostility to the child and also hostile impulses to herself. It should be noted that one of the factors in this patient's illness which undoubtedly led it to continue without adequate care for far too long was the husband's lack of sympathy for his wife and lack of awareness of her emotional state. Because of this the patient received her initial psychiatric treatment in hospital because it was felt that the husband lacked both the ability to assess his wife's progress and the emotional warmth needed to give her sufficient support.

Untreated, many depressions following childbirth will last the usual spell of four to six months. This means the illness beginning in the second to third month will continue until the child is approaching its first birthday. It must be obvious that several months of misery in the home will have a demoralizing effect on the husband and other children and for the whole of this time there is some risk to the mother and her child of hostile outbursts. It should be remembered that any depressed patient presents some measure of suicidal risk. This risk is not necessarily at its greatest when the woman is at her worst. A severely retarded depressive will lack the initiative to do herself any harm and it may be that the risk is greatest as she is becoming depressed—that is at the beginning of the illness—or alternatively just when improvement sets in and she develops sufficient initiative and ability to put into action plans which she had made during her more retarded phase.

As noted, untreated depressive illnesses usually last for some months. With effective treatment, however, the patient may feel perfectly well again within two or three weeks. It is wise to assume, however, that the underlying depressive phase is still there and, if treatment is with the modern drugs, these should usually be maintained for at least two months from the time when the patient appeared to have made a full recovery, and can then be gradually reduced. It is particularly important to note the patient's response to her first menstrual period. It is not uncommon to find that women who have had a depression following childbirth tend to have quite severe pre-menstrual depressive phases. These may precipitate a relapse of the depression and any medication should be continued to cover these phases until it is certain that the patient is free from risks of relapse. This, as in the case of other puerperal illnesses, will often mean some degree of supervision and perhaps treatment for the first year after childbirth.

Some particular mention must be made of the risk of suicide and the method of assessing the risk when suicide is threatened. It is not true to say that patients who threaten suicide do not commit it. Many successful suicides have given clear warning of their intention. Similarly, it is no more true that those who never discuss it are those who are the worst risks. It is never sufficient to rely on the patient's statement alone. The following factors should always be considered. Firstly, the situation in which the threat was made. It may be clearly related to some stress, for example, an unhelpful husband, and clearly related to an attempt to manipulate the environment. In general, a threat to commit suicide implies that the patient has no desire but merely wants to influence other people. Impulses to commit suicide are fairly common and may be quite frightening for the patient who has never previously considered the possibility. They usually imply a fluctuating degree of depression. Most patients who have these impulses are very relieved to be able to discuss them and to know they can have help, or that if the impulse seems overwhelming they can readily get further assistance. For some of these patients a 'phone number to be called in an emergency may literally be life-saving. Ruminations about suicide also require serious consideration. Some women will ruminate about it and then one morning when their depression is at its worst, take desperate action. It is worth remembering that most depressions tend to be worse in the early hours of the morning and the woman who gets up feeling depressed at 4 a.m. to go downstairs to make a cup of tea, may turn the gas on, but fail to light it.

Suicidal ideas, impulses, or preoccupations, should all be taken more seriously in the setting of a sustained depressive mood which has already lasted for more than a few days. If they are associated with depressive delusions, that is feelings of unworthiness, somatic delusions, delusions affecting the baby, these all carry a sinister import. Lastly, and this may be the most significant clue to any immediate risk of suicide, the patient should be asked to discuss her feelings about the future. The patient who refuses to consider the future, or even to discuss it, is unwilling even to consider her activities the next day, may well be considering a way of preventing the next day ever coming for her.

CHAPTER NINE

Psychopathic Personality and Subnormality

(a) Psychopathic Personality

This group of patients includes those who from birth or an early age have shown abnormalities of personality, in particular showing an inability to learn from experience and to modify their way of life so that it is in keeping with the culture and background of their family and local society. Sometimes there is a family history of personality abnormality and there is not uncommonly evidence of alcoholism, criminal behaviour, prostitution or other signs of an abnormal way of life in close relatives. Sometimes this condition appears to be due to the child's upbringing, particularly in its early years and particularly if there has been inconsistency in the standards expected by the parents or parental substitutes. Emotional deprivations in the early years, whatever the cause, may leave the child with impaired ability to form close relationships for the rest of its life. Frequently however the family history will show the child from birth was different in temperament to its siblings and the well-known 'black sheep of the family' is the layman's recognition that a well-ordered and stable family may nevertheless have one anti-social member.

As would be expected, the abnormality of personality produces difficulties in personal relationships from an early age. These children are difficult to rear in the early years and many give a history of temper tantrums or resistance to training before school years. At school there are frequently difficulties with discipline, truancy or other evidence of maladjustment. School reports may comment that the child, although not lacking in intelligence, lacks application or refuses to co-operate in the class. After leaving school there may be multiple changes of job for trivial reasons and not uncommonly overt anti-social acts, leading to a criminal record. As might be expected, promiscuity may begin early and illegitimate pregnancies result. Unfortunately, these patients who frequently have little feeling for others and are largely concerned with their own immediate satisfactions, may use their child to express their own resentment and frustration with other people, rather than adopt a normal maternal attitude towards it.

It is usual to sub-divide the patients with psychopathic personality into three groups. Firstly, those with emotional instability. This type of patient will be well known in her local area because of her explosive emotional tendencies. Following a minor tiff, she may take an overdose or make some other dramatic gesture of despair. If frustrated she may fly into a rage or attack the person concerned. These episodes may be followed by short-lived contrition. Under stable conditions when all goes well, little may appear on the surface to suggest the patient has any abnormality. Her excessive reaction under stress, however, often leads from one crisis to the next. Promises made are quickly forgotten and this type of patient is likely to be one of those who fails to keep out-patient appointments, yet turns up on the wrong day to the inconvenience of all. She may then over-react to minor rebukes. Because of the emotional lability, the child can sometimes be in danger, as in the following case history.

Miss P. was referred by the Health Visitor to her general practitioner because bruises had been found on her child aged one month. Her father had been an alcoholic, often in prison, and when at home liable to terrorize the family. She remembered his rages but had no recollection of any affectionate gesture from him. Her mother had been a dullard who eventually deserted the family, and the patient, together with two siblings, went into the care of the local authority. She remembered creating difficulties at school and frequent truancy. In the home she was noted for her defiance of authority and one attempt at placement in a foster home ended in a month because of her behaviour. She eventually left school and obtained a domestic job but left this without notice to go and live with a casual male acquaintance. At the age of sixteen she had had two miscarriages and for a time lived as a prostitute. When twenty, she developed a more stable relationship though this was with a man with a criminal record for multiple petty offences. He never worked regularly but lived on his wits by casual betting and other borderline social activities. She eventually became pregnant and had a child after living with him for about a year. For the first week or two she appeared fond of her baby and gave it quite a good standard of care and affection. Her 'husband' failed to provide regular financial support and she became increasingly frustrated with him. A careful review of her behaviour showed that when she was annoyed with the man concerned she then hit the baby. This pattern of events recurred on several occasions and by the time the general practitioner was able to visit, a vicious circle of behaviour had been completed. The man concerned was quite fond of his child and upset when the patient hit it. He in turn ill-treated the patient, who waited until his back was turned when she struck the child. Discussion with her showed that she was well aware of the reasons for her actions, aware that other people would consider them wrong though she herself showed no particular guilt or concern. She expressed no desire for treatment for herself but did ask that something should be done for her 'husband' to make sure that he worked regularly. A careful assessment of the domestic situation ensued but, unfortunately, the only result of this was that the 'husband' disappeared and the patient then abandoned her child which had to be taken into local authority care. The patient, too, disappeared for a time, reappearing a month later, tearfully claiming her baby and stating that she never intended to be parted from it again. There was some delay in arranging for reunion and, while waiting, she became sufficiently frustrated with the person making enquiries for a quarrel to develop and she stalked out of the office not to be seen again.

This type of emotional instability tends to become less common with age. Thus, the emotionally unstable psychopath is usually met with in her late adolescence or early adult life. It is rare to meet this type of disability in middle life.

A second group of patients with psychopathic personality includes those with sexual abnormality. No woman is completely feminine any more than any man is completely masculine. Some women, for as long as they can remember, have only had sexual feelings towards their own sex. These are the true homosexuals. Many other women are aware at some phase of their life, particularly in adolescence, of some feeling towards their own sex, though normal heterosexual feelings are also present. For the majority of women, their heterosexual feelings become dominant and heterosexual response is for them the normal occurrence. It might be thought that women with homosexual tendencies only would be unlikely to marry and even more unlikely to have a child. This is not the case. Some women are aware of their homosexual nature but, because of social attitudes despise it, and marry in the hope that they will be cured. Others, perhaps because of a restrictive upbringing, have little awareness of their true nature and marry having given little thought to the sexual side of the relationship. This is particularly likely where the marriage has been 'arranged' by parents or perhaps where the woman has chosen an older man because of his financial or social position but has little true emotional feeling for him. As might be expected, these patients usually restrict their families, and are unlikely to have more than one or two children. They may first appear in the psychiatric clinic because of an unwanted pregnancy, or because their fears of pregnancy have led to major upheavals in the family. They may be conscientious mothers though many of them lack the intuitive feminine touch in baby care. They are likely to prove somewhat matter-of-fact parents, often managing a boy-child better than a girl. It is often tempting to speculate on the possible psychopathology, but if there is a clear history of homosexual tendencies throughout life with no evidence of heterosexual trend at any time, it is unlikely that any form of treatment, psychotherapeutic or otherwise, will alter the situation.

Another group of psychopathic personalities contains those with creative gifts. Many great artists have shown clear evidence of psychopathy, in that throughout their lives, they have had difficulties in personal relationships and some degree of conflict with the society in which they live. Many were men, but artistic traits, together with psychopathy, are by no means uncommon in women too. These women may avoid marriage, regarding it as too conventional, and may become involved in very unusual liaisons. Should pregnancy result, it is common to find that during pregnancy and the puerperium, the woman's previous creative talents are in abeyance. They frequently find child-rearing an inconvenience and will try to arrange for others to act as mother substitute. Their creative gifts will usually return and it is improbable that they will prove very satisfactory mothers in the long run. Those records we have of the home life of children brought up by unstable artists strongly suggest that the woman's tendency to offer child-care to another is in the child's interest as well as her own.

As might be expected, girls with psychopathic tendencies are among these more prone than the average to illegitimate pregnancies. Indeed, the illegitimate pregnancy may be part of the patient's protest against convention and rejection of the advice or standards of those around her. It is this, apart from other considerations, that should make those concerned chary of a termination of pregnancy, merely to solve the immediate problem. The following case history will illustrate the point.

Miss G. came from a good home and was brought up with conventional moral standards. Her parents were both professional people, her mother perhaps a little prudish and restrictive, her father more easy-going and tolerant. The patient was the younger of two girls and, from an early age, showed a tendency to resent and reject the standards of her family. Her elder sister was the more successful and the patient accepted too readily the role of unsuccessful scholar and, later, that of being unsuccessful in her social ambitions. She left school at her own request before taking any examinations and, from her school reports, to the evident relief of her schoolmistresses. Her mother arranged secretarial training but after a few weeks the patient gave this up and went into work as a shop-assistant, giving this up too after a few weeks' trial. She then spent some weeks at home though her parents made it clear they disapproved of her idleness and restricted her pocket-money. She began to adopt extremes of dress and acquired a boy-friend with similar tendencies. She soon quarrelled with him, however, and his place was filled by another equally unsavoury youth. Both of these boys came from families whose standards were far below those of the girl's own parents. She was found to be pregnant and was unable to be sure which of the two boys might be the father. She showed singularly little concern at her difficulties and seemed quite content to stay at home and await the event. Her parents, however, were horrified and eventually persuaded her general practitioner and the local gynaecologist to perform a termination of pregnancy. The futility of this was demonstrated by the fact that the patient became pregnant again within three months, this time by a much older man whom she had met very briefly. He was married and had no intention of forming any permanent relationship with the patient. At this point, she was referred to a psychiatric clinic. At interview she was quite composed and cheerful, readily admitted the facts, and showed no particular concern over her problems. She expressed considerable resentment about the first termination and said she was quite averse to any operations. She admitted she did not really want the child and had made no plans nor given any thought to its future. She was quite pleased with herself and eventually admitted that one of the reasons she had taken no precautions against a further pregnancy was the knowledge that her condition embarrassed her parents and, at least for a time, prevented them from trying to get her to go to work again.

The treatment of a psychopathic personality is very difficult and many consider that the essential nature of the disease makes any formal treatment impossible. Nevertheless, husbands or other relatives will often ask for help or guidance. Although the acute episodes can be managed with symptomatic measures, the personality of the patient will often frustrate any more determined long-term attempts to help her. Some of the tranquillisers do seem to help, particularly those patients with emotional instability, as noted in a later chapter. For the majority, however, the best that can be hoped for is that the patient during her time of crisis will form a relationship with one of her physicians. While her affairs are going well she may refuse appointments and reject advice, but it is often found that if these patients are offered the opportunity of returning for further guidance or support when they are in difficulties, they may make use of these opportunities. Over the years, use of such opportunities to help or support them at times of stress, may prevent some of these patients from creating social disasters in themselves or others, and may help them to live within the framework of society until maturation has occurred. It is essential that all those involved in the social services should be aware of the patient's personality problems and adopt a consistent attitude towards her.

(b) Subnormality

Subnormality is the more modern term for the old diagnosis 'mental deficiency'. By definition this condition begins from birth or an early age. Because of brain damage or shortage of brain tissue the patient is unable to learn and adjust to her environment as would the normal child. The milder degrees of the condition would merely be regarded as dull and backward; the more severe degrees, however, are of such severity that the patient is quite unable to live a normal life and in some cases may never progress beyond the level where total nursing care, including spoon-feeding, is needed. Definitions for two grades of this condition are provided in the Mental Health Act 1959, but it should be remembered that many patients suffer from this condition without at any time in their lives having been diagnosed or treated under the Act.

Severe subnormality means an incomplete development of mind of such a degree that the patient is incapable of living an independent life. On the other hand subnormality under the Act merely means a state of arrested or incomplete development of mind which is of a nature or degree which requires, or is susceptible to medical treatment or other special care or training, of the patient.

Patients suffering from severe subnormality are highly unlikely to become pregnant. Many of course are in hospital. Those at home will need such a degree of care and are so severely handicapped that pregnancy is virtually impossible. Many patients with lesser degrees of subnormality live relatively normal lives. They will have had difficulty at school and may have been to special schools because of their slowness to learn. They can often perform simple work and can earn quite good money in factories or other jobs requiring patience and persistence rather than skill or intellectual ability. Their slowness to learn and faulty judgment however are often revealed by social difficulties. Girls with subnormality can be easily deceived and illegitimate pregnancy is then likely. Emotional instability together with subnormality can lead to severe social difficulties and occasionally repeated illegitimate pregnancies together with a nomadic life, prostitution, or other evidence of social inadequacy is obvious.

Another way in which subnormality presents to the obstetrician is in the patient who appears for the first time in the maternity ward without having had any antenatal examination. Some of these patients are unaware of their rights and entitlement to antenatal care or may be frightened of the complexity of the out-patient organization. They may keep one appointment but then fail to keep others. They are likely to form a considerable proportion of the patients who present as emergencies, either for their own health or that of their babies because of lack of elementary care or normal ante or post-natal precautions. It should be possible to recognize if a patient is of low intelligence and that this will present difficulties from an elementary history of her schooling. Once it is recognized that a degree of subnormality is present, extra care must be taken to ensure adequate ante and post-natal care and a careful personal follow-up by a Social Worker or Health Visitor if any appointment is not kept. Just as extra care will be taken of the patient who has a small pelvis because of the likely complications, so should extra care be taken of the patient who is a dullard. It is no more the fault of the patient with a small pelvis that she has this physical disability than it is of the dullard that from no choice of her own she lacks the judgment and competence of her better endowed sister.

Case history: Miss R., aged 19

Her father was a manual labourer who had many different jobs and was frequently out of work. Her mother was almost illiterate. The patient was the seventh of eight children. As far as the history could be obtained, she failed to walk until she was two and did not talk clearly until nearly four. She had a very poor school record, was frequently away with ill-health and sometimes truanted. She had only reached Standard Four by the age of thirteen and in effect left school at that age in spite of considerable efforts by the Attendance Officer to ensure regular attendance. She could read words of one syllable but did not write more than her own name. She did some domestic work and for some months was a packer in a factory. She was frequently unemployed however. She became pregnant and it was not known by whom. She was taken to the general practitioner by her mother and an antenatal appointment arranged at the local hospital. This she failed to keep. She was next heard of as an emergency when she was admitted to the maternity unit with a massive haemorrhage from a placenta praevia.

The patient's life was saved following a transfusion but the child was born dead.

Subnormality by itself forms inadequate grounds for termination of pregnancy. Dullards can be very affectionate mothers who can give a good standard of care within their limitations. Moreover it must be remembered that their children may well be of higher intelligence than themselves, unless it is known that the subnormality is due to an inherited condition. Nevertheless, subnormality is a considerable handicap and if the patient suffers from other evidence of mental disorder this would add to the factors which would lead a termination to be considered. Similarly, it is obviously more difficult for a woman of low intelligence to manage her own household and bring up her children, and breakdown of one kind or another is more likely under stress. Some subnormal patients find great difficulty in managing any form of contraception and for these there may be a clear indication for sterilization.

CHAPTER TEN

Psychiatric Treatment

(a) General considerations

Treatment of the puerperal psychiatric illness will always involve treatment of the total family. It should be the primary concern of all involved to ensure that the mother/baby relationship is maintained. No hard and fast rule can ever be laid down. Treatment which would be perfectly feasible in the case of the young primipera might be quite impossible in the case of the elderly multipera when one had to consider the total load of responsibility she had to carry. As noted in an earlier chapter, the general practitioner is in a unique position to assess the total family resources and may know not only the patient and her husband and their likely response to stress but may well know the preceding generation too. Although the stress of a psychiatric illness in the puerperium may have considerable repercussions throughout the family there is no doubt that this stress can unite a family just as it may, if mishandled, lead to disorganization.

There are some features of a puerperal psychiatric illness which makes it unique and must be considered in any treatment programme. Firstly, one must consider the impact any treatment, whether pharmacological or psychotherapeutic, will have on the baby as well as the mother. Fortunately, few drugs are excreted through the milk in such quantity that the baby will come to harm. It is likely with most sedatives that an excess at night will make the mother drowsy or clumsy and this, in turn, adds to the risks to her infant. They should always be avoided by day. Secondly, many marked changes in the mental state can occur from day to day, particularly in the first two weeks of the puerperium. This rapid change can be quite misleading. It probably accounts for some of the dramatic cures quoted in the literature and for the remarkably good prognosis given to some conditions by some authors, while others treating those illnesses which have lasted for a longer time found the prognosis more gloomy. It is reassuring for the doctor to hope that a patient who is depressed one day and is well the next is therefore out of danger, but the third day may find a recurrence of the depression, and the fourth a florid schizophrenic psychosis. Even within twenty-four hours there may be quite considerable variations. The patient may appear lucid in the morning to be quite deluded by evening. Lastly, it is common to find that the account given by relatives is considerably distorted by their anxiety. Sometimes it is only the presence of the baby which compels the relatives to take action in an illness of insidious onset. For example, one husband said that his wife had been hallucinated for two years, but he did not worry about it until she had the baby! At this point, he suddenly realized the implication of his wife's symptoms and the possible risks his child might run. Quite commonly the reverse happens and relatives' anxieties have led to a gross exaggeration of the patient's clinical state. For example, they may report that she had threatened to murder the child when the truth is that she put it back in its cradle, saying she could not stand its crying any more.

As in the case of any other illness, an initial assessment of the patient's condition is essential and this should be followed by a further assessment at a short interval. In these particular conditions, one initial impression may be quite misleading. In the early puerperium it is always wise to warn both the patient and her relatives that considerable fluctuations are possible and that changes for neither better nor worse should lead to undue optimism or pessimism. Once some plan has been made for further treatment of the patient and her child, it is absolutely essential that all those involved should be aware of the proposals and adopt a consistent attitude. As noted earlier a considerable number of people are likely to be involved in any one case. Not only the patient, her husband and child, but their parents, occasionally others in the house or close neighbours and of course the medical services, including the general practitioner, Health Visitor and others.

The most important thing of all for the patient is the development of the 'love affair' with her baby. Nothing else will give her so much happiness or satisfaction as the knowledge that this relationship is as perfect as possible. In general it can be said that patients do not need advice in baby-care but merely the provision of the right atmosphere in which baby-care and mother love can develop naturally. It is not uncommon to find that anxious patients have already consulted a number of relatives, a number of books, and sometimes a number of doctors, with no real benefit. Their real need is a peaceful atmosphere, the removal of all other stresses and distractions and the opportunity in quiet privacy to love their own child. There are probably as many ways of baby-management and baby-care as there are mothers. The essential details of baby-washing, nappy-changing, and similar chores are so easily learned that specific advice is very rarely needed, even for the dullard. Each mother will find her own way and the way which suits her and her own child the best. Some guidance may be necessary on the details of artificial feeding but here again within certain limits it is probable that most mothers need the confidence and emotional security to feed their baby adequately, rather than the ability to choose between the niceties of one mixture compared with another. It is well known in large nurseries that babies will flourish on the most simple mixture and the need for special diets is a rarity.

The management of breast-feeding is important. There can be no doubt that for most mothers and babies, breast-feeding is the feeding method of choice. There is no evidence to suggest that a mental illness by itself should lead to a cessation of breast-feeding. The only exception to this rule lies in the toxic psychoses. Here it should be obvious that a woman who is toxic not only may pass this toxaemia to the child through the milk but in her delirium may harm her child. In the acute psychotic disturbances there is no such indication. Most of these mothers will breast-feed their children with success to the baby's obvious benefit and very often to their own obvious emotional relief. If a woman is prevented from breast-feeding, it is likely to confirm her fears that she is failing in her feminine functions and this failure may be reflected in her attitude to the child for the rest of their lives. Many women report that they feel an emotional warmth and closeness for a breast-fed child which they are unable to achieve with one who has been brought up on the bottle. It should be remembered of course that some women are better 'milkers' than others. This frequently runs in the family and is allied to the body-build. Just as it is essential to give a woman her best chance of breast-feeding, in an atmosphere of calm and security, so it is equally important not to make her feel guilty should she fail. The emotional atmosphere around the mother should be one of support whatever her method of feeding may be. The breast of course is a sexual organ and women who can breast-feed successfully are usually those who can accept this fact. The best possible advice to any mother considering breast-feeding is that she should relax and enjoy it. It is certainly important not to produce an atmosphere in which the woman feels she has to 'try'. It is certainly possible for an active baby to obtain a good feed from the mother's breast when the mother is unconscious or in stupor. No active effort on the part of the mother is required. As might be expected, it is the patient with neurotic conflicts about her sexuality and about her own body, who is most likely to find breast-feeding difficult or embarrassing. It is unlikely that the present generation of young women will feel anything like the embarrassment about their own bodies that was felt by the previous generation. In the long run the bikini may do more to encourage breast-feeding than any amount of good advice. A woman who can be proud of her breasts and enjoy them is likely to find pleasure in breast-feeding as well as in other sexual activities. The exception to this rule is the exhibitionistic young lady who may be quite prepared to demonstrate her charms but is reluctant to accept the responsibility or hard work which goes with baby-care.

The maternal instinct does not develop spontaneously in every woman. Some do not develop full maternal feelings until the child is some months or occasionally even a year or two old. There are some women who find it easy to fall in love with a small baby but gradually lose interest as the child becomes a toddler. Other women are the reverse and find young babies difficult and a chore but have immense warmth and sympathy for the toddler. It is tempting to try and trace the reasons for this in the mother's own early life and upbringing. Whatever the reason may be it is important to recognize the possibility. A considerable proportion of women will not feel any spontaneous maternal warmth for their child in the first few days or weeks. They should feel able to discuss this and not feel unduly guilty about it. A very good standard of baby-care is possible even when feelings for the child are limited. Such mothers should be given praise and encouragement for carrying out their maternal duties even when their maternal feelings and drive are limited.

Handling the baby is an essential part of baby-care. Many mothers with their first child treat it as if it were fragile and would break in their hands and there may be some delay before they are able to give spontaneous expression to their feelings and cuddle the child with warmth and vigour. The mother's handling of the child gives many clues to her feelings towards it which she may be unable to verbalize. In general, specific advice on methods of handling should be avoided, as should demonstrations on 'how to do it'. It often helps anxious mothers to have another person present in the room when they are bathing or changing their baby in the first few days. This person, however, should try to avoid comments and criticisms and should merely support the mother, fetch and carry, and generally provide an encouraging background while she is learning how to manage her own child. Each mother/child relationship is unique. This mother must adjust to the reactions of this particular child and the relationship which develops between them should have the minimum of interference from outside.

Sleep presents a problem for many mothers. The lucky ones may have a child which rapidly learns to sleep through the night but, even so, many mothers will find that by the time they have given the child its last feed in the evening and have then completed the chores, they are up again in the morning for the early-morning feed before their full night's sleep has been completed. Most women become very alert to their baby's least sound and this will produce a very light sleep in some. As many of the psychiatric illnesses develop, this light sleep can become severe insomnia. Severe insomnia will lead to further difficulties by day and the increasing tension by day will then affect the possibility of sleep at night. There is then a dilemma in that the patient obviously needs sleep but any heavy sedation will make her heavy-eyed the next morning and may make it impossible for her to care for her child in the night, should he need it. Following childbirth, some patient's reaction to drugs is altered. This too should be born in mind even when a familiar sedative is prescribed. It is important to enquire into the particular difficulty in sleeping and the type of sleep rhythm which has become established. Many women drop off to sleep exhausted but then when the child wakes them at 2 or 3 a.m. find they cannot sleep again. A short-acting sedative given after this night-time feed may be indicated and prove vastly more satisfactory than sedation given earlier in the night. Other women find that they tend to doze and wake throughout the night, never achieving any satisfactory depth of sleep. For these, a short-acting sedative merely produces heavy early sleep but no sleep later in the night. A long-acting sedative such as phenobarbitone may lead to a hangover the next day. In these cases, it will often be found preferable to combine a short-acting sedative with one of the tranquillizers, for example, sodium amylobarbitone grains $1\frac{1}{2}$ to 3 together with chlorpromazine mg. 50 to 100.

The primary cause of any toxic state should be treated, remembering that there is often an increased demand for vitamins, shortage of which can cause psychiatric symptoms. The parenteral route ensures adequate absorption.

(b) Psychotherapy

Psychotherapy can be defined as treatment based on the relationship which develops between people as a result of verbal communication alone. It must be obvious that there will be as many forms of psychotherapy as there are doctors. Each doctor will bring his own unique personality to this situation and the relationship which will develop between him and his patient, or group of patients, will be unique. Nevertheless, it is important to understand the chief forms of psychotherapy which are now in common use. For convenience, these can be subdivided into individual and group psychotherapy and both forms can be subdivided further into these in which emotional support is the chief feature and those in which some form of analysis and change in the psycho-dynamics of the patient are involved.

The old 'bedside manner' contained a considerable element of psychotherapy and most doctors, deliberately or otherwise, cultivated this facet of their treatment. Any doctor will practice individual supportive psychotherapy when he is willing to listen to his patient's problems, discuss them with her, and give her support in her attempts to solve them. Individual analytic psychotherapy however is quite a different matter. This implies an attempt, often over many months or years, to help the patient to understand her relationship with others, at first with the therapist, on the basis of her early life experiences. This form of psychotherapy is likely to cause as well as alleviate anxiety and should not be undertaken except by those who have had training and experience in its use.

It could be said that any group of mothers at a Baby Welfare Clinic will practise supportive group psychotherapy. They will certainly discuss their common problems and encourage each other in methods of baby-care and help relieve the common minor anxieties which each will experience. In an out-patient clinic or day-hospital setting, groups of young mothers may meet to discuss common problems and be helped by discussion in the presence of a sympathetic and helpful doctor to face common difficulties. Other groups, however, can be formed with young mothers, together perhaps with their husbands or other patients in which the most important feature is an attempt to understand the patient's personality and interaction with other people. An attempt can be made to alter long-term personality difficulties. This type of group psychotherapy does not necessarily need a psycho-analytic background or training in the case of the doctors in charge. Nevertheless, there are some risks in group psychotherapy of this kind which should discourage the inexperienced from starting a group unless they have the support and guidance of someone with considerable past experience.

A better understanding of the forms of psychotherapy may be obtained if we consider their use and application to one particular case.

For example, Mrs K.

She complained that following childbirth she had become lacking in confidence, fearful of going out, shy of meeting strangers, and prone to tears with little stress. She gave the following history: her mother was a fussy, over-anxious woman, somewhat possessive and tending to dominate her household. The patients' father was a kindly, somewhat inadequate man who showed relatively little interest in his children, and gave in to his wife's over-anxiety and tendency to over-organize the household. The patient was the elder of two sisters by four years. She considered that she had had a happy life at home and had been well cared-for by her parents. She had tended to prefer her mother during her school-days and had been somewhat tied to the latter's apron-strings. In adolescence however she began to rebel a little against her mother's over-anxiety and noticed at this stage of her life that her father showed her relatively little affection. She was slow to make boy-friends and only married when she was 24. Initially, there was difficulty in the sexual adjustment though, by the time she became pregnant a year later, she was able to obtain some enjoyment from it. Pregnancy was uneventful and the patient breast-fed her baby for the first two weeks but soon after her return home from hospital weaned the child to the bottle. Her symptoms began within a month of returning home and the patient sought treatment a month later.

Supportive psychotherapy may be given by the general practitioner, by the psychiatrist, or by the gynaecologist in the post-natal clinic. All will need to assess the patient's background, upbringing, personality and present stresses. In general, it is unwise to give advice. If advice is given, the patient may come to rely on this to solve a number of her difficulties and this could tend to produce a dependent relationship on the person giving the advice. Since the object of all psychotherapy is to enable a patient to mature, to develop her own potential, and to solve her own problems, the encouragement of a dependent relationship must frustrate this. The patient should be helped to feel that any suggestions *she* may make will be welcomed and that she will be supported in any attempts she makes herself to improve the situation. Questions which give some suggestions to her are better than direct advice. For example, this patient has fears of going out. Rather than urge her to try again, it is better to discuss with her the occasions on which she does go out, whether she and her husband have been able to get away from their household chores together and whether she can easily get baby-sitters. In this type of psychotherapy, little attempt is made to delve into the reasons for her fears, other than forthright enquiry as to any anxieties she may have. On the other hand, she is encouraged to ventilate any fears or conflicts and when necessary is reassured, particularly if she has difficulties common to many women in her situation. The most important aspect of this form of treatment is that the patient should feel that there is someone who will be on her side, will support her in difficulties, will give her encouragement in her own attempts to widen her own experience or improve her performances, whether it be in baby-care, in her relationship with her husband or her relationship with the outside world.

Individual analytic therapy would involve a very different approach. In formal psychoanalysis the patient would need to give an hour a day, five days a week, for two or three years, if a whole and formal treatment were to be completed. Nowadays, a number of analysts are trying shorter methods of treatment, sometimes involving a matter of months. In some cases there has been the use of drugs and abreactive or hypnotic techniques to shorten the process. The difficulties involved in formal psychoanalysis in the case of a woman with a young baby and the usual ties to the home this represents, are considerable. Nevertheless, if this method is recommended, it can be assumed that the patient in the process of analysis will begin to bring to the analytic session evidence of her past emotional problems and conflicts. In the case of the particular woman we are considering it is likely that quite early in the analysis she will complain that the analyst was not helping her enough or giving her sufficient attention. If, as we are assuming, the analyst is a man, it is likely that this will be interpreted as a response to him as a father figure; just as she felt her own father did not give her sufficient care, so she now feels the analyst is responding in the same way. As the analysis proceeds it is likely that the patient would find and be guided to find by her analyst similar feelings towards other people in her life based on her early life experience. Some people in her life might represent her mother and her mother's over-anxious dominating attitudes. There is no doubt in the case of the young mother that she would find in the course of treatment that she tended either to reproduce her mother's attitudes towards her own child or, on other occasions, the reverse of these attitudes when they had been rejected. Other possibilities in the case quoted would include the likelihood, if her own baby was a girl, that she might feel considerable jealousy and resentment over this child. It is likely in her early life that, when her sister was born, she, who had been the only child for four years, felt considerable resentment and jealousy. Now, in her own adult life, when she has her own baby girl, she may fear loss of affection from her husband or others in the environment who might give preference to the newcomer. In the case history, it was noted that the patient had some difficulty in sexual adjustment. If we assume that she was an inhibited woman who perhaps had chosen a relatively dull and unadventurous man, the experience of childbirth may well have altered her emotional responses. She may now find herself much more easily aroused and with much more sexual feeling than before. Her husband may appear relatively dull and uninteresting and she may be frightened by her own sexual response to other men. This is one possible explanation of her fears of going out. It can be seen that the emotional content of a psychoanalysis is very much more personal and likely to be much more emotionally disturbing to the patient. Some of it she would certainly reject in the ordinary way and may only be able to accept it as being part of her own personality and problems following considerable preparation in the analytic process.

Supportive group psychotherapy is readily organized in the out-patient clinic, day-hospital, or even in the post-natal clinic. Young mothers tend to support each other by a natural 'instinct'. The more extroverted and sociable will certainly talk of their difficulties freely and exchange information about changes, attitudes, and common problems. It is the shy and the inhibited (and these traits often go with neurosis) who tend to be left out of the very conversations which might relieve their anxieties. Many supportive out-patient groups consist of the more shy and isolated young mothers in a neighbourhood and these young mothers will find very considerable benefit by a discussion, particularly with some guidance and help from the doctor. As with individual supportive psychotherapy, this type of group will encourage the young mother to ventilate her problems, to discuss her background and difficulties, and the group as a whole will support each individual member in attempts to overcome emotional difficulties or fears. In some cases, there is no doubt that a patient can accept suggestions or try to follow out advice given by a group of people with similar background, better than she can from a doctor who, if he is a man, she may regard as something of an outsider in this particular situation.

In a group which aims at some analysis of personality traits and attitudes, there will be a different approach. These groups may consist of young mothers only but, sometimes, will be more effective if there is a mixture of patients, some of whom may be mothers, some single, and some men too present. It is an advantage if those in the group are roughly of similar intelligence and have a similar type of problem, i.e. a neurosis as opposed to a psychosis, or psychopathic personality. It should be made clear at the outset that the function of a group is to reveal personality traits and attitudes and, if each group member is to obtain some personal benefit, each must play their part in helping the others to understand their reactions, tolerate each other's difficulties, and support each other in attempts to change. If we take our patient, we might find a group for her where there are a number of young women, one or two older ones, and one or two men of varying ages. We will find our young mother reluctant to speak or discuss her problems. She will probably tend to seek support from an older woman in the group and similarly tend to assume that the older men in the group would show little interest in her. At some point, other group members would notice this and raise it for discussion and try to find the reasons for it. As the group progressed it might become apparent that, as well as looking for support from an older woman in the group, the patient also resented this older person's advice when given and any evidence she showed of trying to help. Here again, a group would enable the patient to realize that those feelings are those she had towards her own mother. It is very likely that at some point the patient's feelings towards her own child would be discussed and her own attitude towards motherhood, based on her own early life experience would be revealed. Within the group it may be possible for her to try and become more mature, more certain of herself as a woman and of her own ability to live her own life without being bound by attitudes inculcated by her mother. Confidence in herself, developed in the group situation, should enable her to overcome the lack of confidence she has shown in her relationships since the birth of her child.

(c) *Physical treatment*

Fifty years ago there were no effective physical treatments in psychiatry other than the crudest sedation. Today there is such a plethora of drugs and physical treatments of all kinds that the newcomer to this side of psychiatry may well be bewildered by their diversity. There are now some dozens of tranquillizers in everyday use and almost a dozen anti-depressants with which most physicians will have some acquaintance. It is important in this sphere of medicine as in any other that the physician should become familiar with the effects and side-effects of a small range of drugs rather than try a very wide variety and fail to become familiar with any one of them. There is one particular aspect of drug therapy which is of considerable significance for psychiatry and which plays a relatively small part in the rest of medicine. There can be no doubt that some drugs seem to work for some physicians better than for others. It can happen that a drug prescribed by one physician fails to produce any effect but when the same dosage is prescribed by another, obvious changes occur. There is at least one obvious explanation for this phenomenon. For example, if we have a drug with stimulant effect, prescribed by a physician who himself tends to take an energetic role in the doctor/patient relationship and by his manner and comments clearly expects the patient to be stimulated, the drug, because of its innate action together with the suggestions from the physician, is likely to stimulate. The same drug prescribed by a physician whose attitude is more passive and who may by his comments and suggestions lead the patient to expect some measure of relaxation rather than stimulation, may have little or no effect, even in the same dosage. The influence of the physician's expectations is more obvious in psychiatric treatment than in any other sphere of medicine.

The drugs in common use can be subdivided into the sedatives, the stimulants, the tranquillizers, and the anti-depressants. Anti-convulsants are used by psychiatrists, neurologists and physicians for those patients with epilepsy, and will not be considered in further detail here. The treatment of epilepsy is in no way different in pregnancy and the puerperium than at any other time and it is notoriously difficult to predict whether pregnancy and the puerperium will have any effect whatever on the incidence of fits. Caution with any new drug is essential in the first three months of pregnancy.

Sedatives. Before any sedatives are prescribed, it is essential to consider whether they are necessary or not, particularly for some condition which is likely to be temporary. Current evidence suggests that the effect of even a few nights' sedation is prolonged far beyond the effect on those particular nights. Many patients who have taken sedatives for a week for some temporary condition have found it has taken twice that period to regain a normal sleep rhythm without them. Many patients have become minor addicts as a result of sedation. Nevertheless, it is important for a woman under stress to have adequate sleep, otherwise her mental health will certainly suffer and it is notorious that a few severely disturbed nights are liable to precipitate both anxiety and depressive reactions. There is one situation in particular where adequate sedation seems essential. This is during the first few nights immediately after childbirth. Many women find that the stress and excitement of child-bearing is so intense that memories of it prevent sleep for the first few nights after the event. They may relive their experiences, whether pleasurable or unpleasurable; memories and phrases float up in the mind as they try to drop off to sleep and this can cause very considerable distress. Any woman with this experience should be able to obtain sufficient night sedation to help her to achieve sleep. This condition is an excellent example of one which will usually respond to a short-acting sedative such as sodium amytal. Phenobarbitone should be avoided because of its prolonged action; often such a large dose will be needed to ensure early sleep that far more will be given than is strictly needed for the purposes of the total night. Sodium barbitone is another sedative which used to be very popular but has fallen into disuse. This particular sedative is of little value in those patients who have difficulty in getting off to sleep but can be valuable for those who find they wake in the early hours and then cannot get to sleep again. As noted earlier it is usually preferable to give a short-acting sedative together with chlorpromazine to prolong its effect.

In general, day-time sedation should be avoided. There is little doubt that those patients who take day-time sedatives in any quantity usually need a larger dose at night to achieve sleep. This is the setting *par excellence* for producing a degree of addiction. Moreover, in the puerperium a drowsy mother is a positive danger to her infant. In the past, it may have been necessary to prescribe sedatives for young mothers, but under present conditions, with a wide choice of tranquillizers which have minimal sedative effects, such old-fashioned prescribing is no longer justifiable. Each physician will have his own preference among the short-acting sedatives for night-time use. Among the more recent which are of value should be mentioned nitrazepam. It should be avoided early in pregnancy. This compound is allied to chlordiazipoxide which is more commonly used as a minor tranquillizer during the day, though this too can be quite a useful mild night sedative given as one or two capsules.

The anti-depressant drugs of the past, such as benzedrine, are more correctly termed stimulants. It is only in the last ten years that the true anti-depressants have been available. The first of these was imipramine. It is a useful drug for the milder depressions in the puerperium, though it does have some significant side-effects. The most important of these is the result of its hypotensive action. All patients should be warned to take imipramine when they have food in the stomach and should be warned that otherwise they may feel dizzy or even faint. It is often wise to commence treatment with 10 mgm. three times a day for a day or two to assess the patient's reaction, then increasing every other day to 25 mg. three times a day, then 50 mg. three times a day, and then 50 mg. four times a day. Further increases are possible, but it is rarely necessary to give more than one hundred milligrams four times a day, and the majority of patients will respond to half this dose. It usually leads to some improvement in the mood, an increased appetite and a reduced emotional lability. Some patients complain of increased sweating and, occasionally, a generalized dermatitis can occur. Serious blood dyscrasias or liver damage are very rare. There are other drugs based on the same chemical structure as imipramine, which seem to show little significant improvement, although claims have been made that they are more quickly acting.

Amitriptyline has very similar effects to imipramine. It does however have a greater tendency to produce some slight sedative effect and this can on occasion be useful. Hypotension is less marked and excessive perspiration and skin rashes less common. On the other hand, some patients do complain of digestive disturbance and also of some muscular inco-ordination. Of the two drugs, imipramine is usually the better tolerated in the puerperium and there is nothing to choose between the two during pregnancy. Both drugs produce their effects slowly. In the case of patients taking imipramine, benefits may not be apparent for at least two weeks, amitriptyline rather more quickly—effects are usually apparent at the end of the first week.

The mono-amine-oxidase inhibitors have received a great

deal of publicity and, when initially introduced, appeared to have very considerable advantages and their side-effects were believed to be minimal. Further experience has shown both beliefs to be wrong. Their side-effects can be very serious including sudden death. Patients have to be given specific warning about their diet while on these drugs and they are also incompatible with a considerable variety of other active drugs in particular the amphetamines, imipramine, anaesthetics and other drugs affecting the nervous system. It is particularly important to warn all patients of the nature of the drug they are taking and its incompatibility with some foodstuffs, particularly cheese, broad beans and Marmite, and that they should warn any doctor treating them for any other condition of the drug they have been taking. It can be seen at once that patients who are already perhaps depressed and anxious may be considerably more so at the knowledge they are taking such a potentially dangerous drug. Of those available, tranylcypromine in a dosage of 10 mg. morning and midday increased to 20 mg. morning and midday often acts as effectively as any. In some patients, it does seem to have a similar stimulant effect as would be expected with the amphetamine group but, fortunately, does not lead to any of the 'hangover' common in the amphetamines. Addiction however is possible. Because of the stimulant effect however, some patients find it more difficult to obtain sleep and need a night sedative while taking the drug. It should not be taken late in the day.

It should be remembered that with any effective anti-depressant therapy, there is always some risk of the precipitation of a manic episode. This is much more likely in the patient with a previous history of a manic episode but can occasionally occur in a patient with no previous history nor with any previous warning. The three anti-depressant drugs mentioned are perhaps typical of their class. Each doctor, as previously noted, may develop his own preference for another member of the group. In general, however, it will be found that it is safest to try drugs roughly in the order suggested, giving some preference to imipramine, later amitriptyline and, if further attempts seem justified, one of the mono-amine-oxidase-inhibitors. It must be remembered however that patients who feel that drugs are being 'tried out' on them, may lose faith in their doctor and tend to resent suggestion of further 'pill medication'.

The tranquillizers. Chlorpromazine was the first tranquillizer in use and is still, in many situations, the first tranquillizer of choice, particularly in the acutely disturbed psychotic patient, whether the psychosis is functional as in schizophrenia or mania, or organic as in delirium and toxic states. A trivial dosage, such as 25 mg. t.d.s. may be ill-tolerated by the patient with a neurosis. This type of patient frequently complains excessively of the side-effects of chlorpromazine. The more disturbed psychotic however may tolerate very large doses, up to 1,000 mg. three times a day. An ordinary dose for a disturbed schizophrenic patient will be 100 to 200 mg. three times a day. Physical frailty is not necessarily a contra-indication to large doses of chlorpromazine. Very frail patients weighing no more than six or seven stone may tolerate several hundred milligrams three times a day and remain alert and co-operative as a result.

Thioridazine is another major tranquillizer which can be used an alternative to chlorpromazine if the latter is not tolerated. The dosage is similar except that thioridazine should not be used above a dosage of 400 mg. three times daily. Trifluoperazine is used in much smaller dosage and is effective if given twice a day. One milligram to two milligrams twice a day often give a measure of symtomatic relief to patients suffering from anxiety states and in particular seems to reduce the somatic side-effects of anxiety. It is also useful in psychoses but in schizophrenia a much larger dose is indicated—5 mg. to 20 mg. twice daily. This dosage is likely to produce Parkinsonian side-effects and it is therefore more usual to give 5 mg. to 15 mg. three times daily together with orphenadrine 50 mg. three times daily. This drug is often more useful than chlorpromazine in schizophrenic patients who present with lethargy rather than excitement.

Haloperidol is used in psychotic patients chiefly to treat states of excitement and is sometimes dramatically effective in mania. The usual dosage is 1·5 mg. to 3 mg. three times daily. This drug too tends to produce the Parkinsonian syndrome sufficiently frequently that orphenadrine or other similar drugs should be given with it.

There is a very large number of tranquillizers and, as emphasized previously, it is better for the practitioner to become familiar with one or two rather than try the effects of many indiscriminately. All of them have side-effects, occasionally serious. The side-effects of each must be known and in particular it is important to know when the side-effects tend to summate or cancel each other out. For example, chlorpromazine and trifluoperazine are often prescribed together and Parkinsonian symptoms due to trifluoperazine are then rare. It is striking that a patient who has Parkinsonian symptoms from trifluoperazine may get dramatic relief from an intra-muscular injection of chlorpromazine. On the other hand chlorpromazine and imipramine both lower the blood pressure and, if prescribed together, may cause severe dizziness and fainting in some patients.

Lastly, it should be remembered that many anti-depressants and tranquillizers are only effective if given over a considerable period; for example, many anti-depressants produce little effect until the patient has taken them in appropriate dosage for a week or two. Equally, once the patient is improving it is often necessary to maintain the dosage for two or three months. Throughout this time the patient should be under medical supervision at regular intervals. This must mean that each time the physician prescribes he should remember that he will need to maintain and supervise medication for several months and should consider whether the patient's illness is of such severity as to justify this.

Electro-convulsive therapy (E.C.T.). The induction of an epileptic fit was first suggested on empirical grounds in that there seemed to be very few patients with epilepsy who later developed schizophrenia. It was thought therefore that there was some antithesis between the two diseases. Initially, the fit was induced by chemical means but it was soon found that electricity was safer, pleasanter for the patient and more precise in its application. Moreover, it was soon found that convulsive therapy produced relief more commonly in patients with depressive illnesses than in those with schizophrenia. In spite of the large number of drugs now available, E.C.T. continues to hold a major place in the psychiatric armamentarium. No other treatment is quite so effective in the acutely disturbed psychotic, in the depressive who is a severe suicidal risk, or the acutely disturbed patient with schizophrenia.

There are several specific considerations during pregnancy and the puerperium. Firstly, during pregnancy the vulnerability of the foetus to anoxia must be remembered particularly in the first few months. Nowadays, when it is usual to modify the fit with a muscle-relaxant, particular care should be taken to see that the patient is fully oxygenated before, during, and after the fit. It is probably better to avoid E.C.T. during the first three months, particularly at the times when miscarriage is most likely, that is at the time when the monthly period would have occurred. In the middle three months, E.C.T. seems very safe and there is very little evidence to suggest that E.C.T. in the last three months is likely to precipitate childbirth. In the puerperium, there is a specific risk in that pulmonary embolism can occur if fragments of thrombi are dislodged from veins which have become thrombosed in the pelvis or legs. Obviously known thrombo-phlebitis would be a contra-indication to E.C.T. but sometimes in the puerperium venous thromboses have formed silently and a disaster may occur without warning. A survey of the literature, however, suggests that the risk of embolism with E.C.T. is small and, moreover, most of the recorded cases have occurred when E.C.T. has been given with a muscle-relaxant. Because of this and for other reasons the author never uses a muscle-relaxant, except in a case of recent fracture or other positive indication, when giving E.C.T. in the puerperium. In over a thousand treatments, many of them given in the first two weeks of the puerperium, there have been no embolic phenomena and no deaths, as a result of E.C.T. given 'straight'.

E.C.T. is indicated in any endogenous depressions where there is some immediate suicidal risk or where the illness has failed to respond to other measures. Most of the anti-depressants take two to three weeks to produce their full effect. It is obviously unwise to allow a woman with clear suicidal intentions to take drugs and await improvement. Even with skilled care and good observation, a patient who has determined suicidal intentions, may well succeed. Similarly, assuming there is some risk of suicide in every depressive illness, it is unwise to try one drug and then another and perhaps a third on the assumption that the patient's illness is sufficiently mild that the risk of self-harm is small. A patient who has had several trials of drugs may become so disheartened and have such little faith in her own chance of recovery and in the ability of her doctor to help her, that she may make some desperate gesture of despair. In general, it can be said that the depressive illnesses of such severity that delusions are present will usually be best treated with E.C.T. For woman who say that their condition is quite hopeless, there is no future for them, that they would be better dead, their child is abnormal or deformed, that they have some awful illness, or make similar delusional statements, E.C.T. should be considered the treatment of choice. E.C.T. can now be made available on an in-patient or out-patient basis, and breast-feeding is in no way contra-indicated. With the present short-acting sedatives or, indeed, if E.C.T. is given 'straight', breast-feeding is possible within half an hour of the treatment. It should be remembered that a healthy baby can obtain a good meal even if the mother is unconscious and, occasionally, in a severely disturbed patient it may be convenient to arrange for the baby to have a meal at the breast before the mother has recovered from her E.C.T. The author has given twenty or more

E.C.T. to mothers who have successfully breast-fed their babies throughout. In general, the depressive illnesses respond quickly to E.C.T. There may be fairly obvious improvement after the first one or two. It is rarely necessary to give more than half a dozen. A considerable number of depressive illnesses however tend to recur, particularly within the first few months of treatment and also, particularly, at the pre-menstrual time. For these relapses, it may be found that a very short course of the treatment—perhaps two or three—will be sufficient for relief, whereas the initial illness did need half a dozen.

The use of E.C.T. in schizophrenia is less clear-cut than in the depressive illnesses. As previously noted, many patients with schizophrenia are relatively well during pregnancy, though symptoms of the illness may reappear during the last month before childbirth. It is usual to manage the symptoms at this stage with tranquillizers. In the puerperium however there is an unusually good opportunity to treat the patient with schizophrenia, in the hope of achieving a higher level of improvement than previously possible. It seems likely that the emotional lability of the early puerperium does provide a situation where treatment may be more effective than at other times. There is also evidence to suggest that the presence of the baby gives the patient with schizophrenia a fresh motive for recovery, a fresh link with reality, and a fresh emotional drive to overcome the handicap of her illness. It is certainly striking that some patients with schizophrenia seem to have a fresh lease of emotional life, with their baby, even though in other respects, their illness may be worse. It is particularly important therefore to treat the patient *with* her child, irrespective of the method used. Some experts would restrict the use of E.C.T. to those patients where the onset has been recent and under stress. This particular group is the group which will tend to recover with or without treatment. In the author's experience, many patients with schizophrenia, even the hebephrenic and occasionally the simple type, will respond to E.C.T. given at this time. There is also some difference of opinion on the number of E.C.T. which should be used in any particular case. Some writers advise the use of frequent E.C.T. until the florid symptoms have been relieved, when tranquillizing drugs will be used instead. This policy is often effective with a recent case of good prognosis but it is notorious that this policy leads to a very high relapse rate in those patients where the illness is of long duration or there is evidence of significant emotional flattening or deterioration. In the author's experience, once a patient with schizophrenia has failed to respond to tranquillizers and has become sufficiently ill to be admitted to mental hospital, it is likely that much more E.C.T. will be needed than merely the few to relieve the acute symptoms. It is his own practice to give approximately twenty and sometimes more in the more resistant cases of schizophrenia. If treatment is given daily, until the acute symptoms have subsided and then at the rate of three a week for three or four weeks, later reducing to two a week and then one a week for the last few treatments, surprisingly good results can be obtained in apparently hopeless cases. E.C.T. given frequently in young patients, i.e. given daily for a week, causes less confusion than might be expected. If however E.C.T. is given three times weekly as outlined, in the third and fourth weeks some confusion is to be expected and some memory loss for these weeks will be persistent. It has been shown however that with a full course of treatment to a total of twenty over approximately two months there will be no effective memory loss for day-to-day events within a week of treatment being completed. It is very rare indeed to find schizophrenic symptoms persisting during the confusion caused by E.C.T. and, once this latter confusion clears, the patient will often be found to have regained her affect and initiative. Flattening of affect and loss of initiative often tend to persist when tranquillizers alone are used.

Hormones. The large drop in circulating hormone levels between pregnancy and the puerperium has already been described. Many studies have shown that the hormone levels are often abnormal in a woman with a psychiatric illness. In the author's experience these abnormalities have not correlated either with diagnosis, severity of illness or the clinical state. In general hormone levels return to normal as the patient improves, but therapeutic efforts to interfere with this process have often proved unsatisfactory. There are two hormones however which warrant further discussion, thyroxine and progesterone.

The thyroid gland shows increased activity during pregnancy, but the amount of circulating hormone rapidly falls after childbirth and, in many women, reaches a relatively low level within a week or two of childbirth, and a normal level may not be regained for several months. Thyroid extract or, preferably, thyroxine are of value in three syndromes. Firstly, there are a number of women who find that, although breast-feeding is well established milk flow diminishes after a few weeks. In some cases there is dramatic improvement when thyroxine is given. Physiology text-books record the importance of the thyroid in the maintenance of lactation, but this information does not seem so readily available elsewhere. Secondly, many women find that between the second and the sixth month after childbirth they feel relatively sluggish, with dry hair, a lack of spontaneity, some constipation, and a tendency to put on weight. Sometimes their hairdresser will comment on the lack of 'life' in their hair. This syndrome is easily confused with a mild depression or simply attributed to the stress and strain of baby-care. In mild degree biochemical changes may be slight and a simple therapeutic trial may be of greater value than extensive testing. In the author's experience biochemical tests in this situation are of limited value; when they are obviously abnormal the clinical diagnosis is equally easy. Considerable fluctuations, however, in all hormone levels occur in the first few weeks of the puerperium and unless the patient's previous levels are known the relevance of the new ones is in doubt. Considerable abnormalities often seem compatible with good health and sometimes only minor abnormalities appear in the tests when there is obvious clinical disability.

The third syndrome, which is often dramatically cured with thyroxine, is frigidity. Frigidity can have many causes, including of course the pain from local disease, simple loss of interest from fatigue, and the normal withdrawal of interest during breast-feeding. Many women recommence sexual relations within a few weeks of childbirth, in order to keep their husband's interest, or to prove their own normality again. Many, however, find that their interest disappears completely for some months. This may lead to no difficulty in some families but in others will be a serious source of distress. Thyroid hormone certainly increases responsiveness. Many women will find that thyroxine in small dosage for a few months will enable them to enjoy their married life and reduce tensions in the household.

Although there have been a number of claims for treatment by progesterone or progesterone-like substances clinical experience is not so clear-cut as in the case of thyroid. It has been suggested that puerperal depressions in particular respond to progesterone and there is some evidence that this hormone has a euphoriant action in some women. It has also been used for those recurrent depressions which are precipitated in the premenstrual phase. Unfortunately pre-menstrual tension is so variable in degree and responds to such a variety of treatments that it is often difficult to prove that any one remedy is essential. Those who claim benefits from the use of progesterone emphasize the need for a large dose.

CHAPTER ELEVEN

Termination and Sterilization

There can be no other subject in medicine which arouses such strong feelings as the question of termination of pregnancy. Sincere men can hold completely contrasting views and this applies not only to those with strong religious convictions. There are those who would argue that termination of pregnancy is equivalent to murder and is never justified. Others, on the other hand, would argue that to bear an unwanted child is in itself such a potential evil that a termination of pregnancy at the simple request of the woman concerned should be made legal. As in most subjects the majority of psychiatrists, gynaecologists and physicians, tend to take a view somewhere between these two extremes. Even the precise interpretation of the legal position is in doubt and the subject of argument. Some would argue that termination of pregnancy is only justified if it is certain that the mother's life or health would be forfeited otherwise. Others, quoting the Bourne case, would suggest that evidence that the mother's mental health *might* be permanently affected is sufficient. Yet others would suggest that such evidence to suggest the mother's mental or physical health might be in some measure the worse would be insufficient grounds. Unfortunately, though some facts and many varying opinions can be found, there is not available at present sufficient evidence of a reliable kind in any series of cases (including control groups) to show whether termination does more good than harm. Moreover, even if reliable figures for different groups of patients were available, each patient is unique in her own history and present stress. It is essential therefore to consider each case upon its merits, knowing that the mental health of some women *does* suffer permanent damage as a result of childbearing.

Most doctors feel aversion to a termination of pregnancy. In view of their training and experience, they are aware that it does mean ending a potential life. It must be remembered that the law (at present) does not sanction termination of pregnancy simply because the child itself might or will be born deformed. In recent years there has been some tendency to accept termination of pregnancy on the grounds that the mother will be mentally disturbed should she give birth to a deformed infant, for example, a 'thalidomide baby'. Although this has been accepted in some cases, the law as it stands does not justify termination on the grounds of the potential abnormality in the child. Some patients threaten that if termination is not done legally, they will go to a back-street abortionist and then any harm they suffer will be the 'fault' of the practitioner who refused operation. This form of blackmail must be resisted. A decision concerning termination of pregnancy is always a serious one, affecting for good or ill, the health and future of the woman concerned. Moreover, the decision by itself does not end the problem. Whether or no she has the child, she will certainly require further psychiatric care and supervision. *If* the risks of psychiatric disturbance are so great that termination is justified, it is quite certain that the risks of some further breakdown, following operation or following other stress in the near future, may also lead to breakdown. No psychiatrist should recommend or surgical team perform the operation and then feel that the problem is solved. Moreover only by further thorough supervision will it be possible to obtain accurate statistics on the future health and welfare in these patients. Many people now consider that it is better to have what has been called a 'termination panel' to decide in all cases where termination is requested. Usually, this board or panel would consist of the patient's practitioner, the psychiatrist concerned and the gynaecologist who will perform the operation. These three must know that any good or ill effects will be their responsibility and, between them, they will have to provide any further treatment she may need for further physical or psychiatric disability. It is always a mistake for a patient needing termination to be seen for this one incident of her life by a different general practitioner, a different psychiatrist and a strange gynaecologist. Only those who will carry the burden of the consequences of termination should recommend or carry it out.

Since we are considering psychiatric disorders it will rapidly become obvious that the patient's own complaints or symptoms by themselves should not be accepted as a basis for action. For example, a patient with long-standing schizophrenic illness who has become pregnant by a casual acquaintance may complain of no symptoms, make no reference to her pregnancy, and make no request for termination. Yet in this case there may be strong grounds for suggesting that the operation should take place. On the other hand, a recently married and emotional young girl may find herself pregnant and resent it, as she had planned to postpone pregnancy for two or three years. She may loudly threaten suicide unless a termination is performed, but since these threats may take place during the early months of emotional lability little weight should be given to them unless there is other strong evidence suggestive of mental illness. No termination on psychiatric grounds should be performed without the fullest assessment, not only of the patient's present mental state, but her background and previous history, home environment and total resources.

We will consider the individual illnesses. The functional psychoses are precipitated by childbearing sufficiently frequently that most psychiatrists believe that a history of recurrent psychosis of this type would form grounds for a termination in any further pregnancy. Even here, however, the total situation of the family and the present family resources, should be considered before any sudden decision is made. The evidence is clearest in the case of schizophrenia. There can be no doubt that for any woman who has had a schizophrenic illness at any time in her life, there is very real risk of relapse in the months following the birth of a child. This relapse may be more severe or less severe than in the original illness and may differ from it in type. Nevertheless, in a personal series it was found that those women who had had a schizophrenic illness of sufficient severity to justify a period of treatment in a mental hospital, further childbearing led to some measure of relapse in the majority. Moreover, this relapse seemed unpredictable. It was as likely to occur in a woman who had made a very good recovery and had an excellent supportive home as in a patient left with some measure of personality deterioration and a difficult home background.

It is particularly difficult in the case of those patients who have found that their schizophrenic symptoms tend to be relieved by pregnancy. These women may welcome a pregnancy because of the relief they feel and lack of insight may prevent them from realizing the serious risk they run of further deterioration in the puerperium. One example of this was a woman who had developed schizophrenia in adolescence and made a partial recovery. She then had an illegitimate pregnancy, during which she felt relatively well but had a further relapse after the baby was born. At this point, she met a man who was illiterate and borderline subnormal and proceeded to have a series of pregnancies by him. By the time a full assessment of her condition was made she had six living children, all of them in the care of the local authority. She lived with her husband who was unemployable and in the last ten years has spent more of her time pregnant than otherwise.

If the patient has had one schizophrenic illness and has made a good recovery, although there is considerable risk that she will have a relapse after childbearing this by itself would not justify a termination. If, for example, the patient has a stable home, a reliable husband, and all other factors are satisfactory, it is probable that even if she has another schizophrenic illness a satisfactory recovery can be expected with modern treatment. If, on the other hand, the patient has had one schizophrenic illness and now has an illegitimate pregnancy and will lack the support of her parents quite a different attitude can be adopted. It may be suspected that the illegitimate pregnancy may itself stem from some lack of judgment or personality defect left from the original illness. Moreover, the combination of schizophrenia and an illegitimate child carries a bad prognosis. Not uncommonly these patients do try to keep their children and there is an endless succession of relapses under the stress, frequent partings, miserable reunions, and eventually the child is lost to someone else's care and the patient left with permanent personality deterioration.

If the patient has had one schizophrenic illness, perhaps after a third child, and is now pregnant with a fourth, much will depend on the total family constellation whether the risk of a further child is justified. There is the risk of a further schizophrenic illness with the disruption to the total family unit this will entail. A schizophrenic illness will often mean the patient leaving home for a month or two and being handicapped for several months more. Even if she can take her baby with her to a Mother and Baby Unit the rest of the family will certainly suffer. Moreover there is, with schizophrenia, the risk of some permanent personality deterioration after every acute episode. For example, a patient had a schizophrenic illness after her first child but made an excellent recovery. She had a second child without relapse or any significant symptom or problem. She became pregnant with her third child and felt very well for the first seven months but began to feel depressed and uneasy in the latter months of pregnancy. A fortnight after the child was born she had a further florid schizophrenic illness. This responded slowly to treatment and a full recovery never occurred. Eventually the patient was able to return home from mental hospital but her adjustment was precarious. She was able to manage her domestic life, but never able again to take the care of *any* of her children.

Sometimes the pregnancy is the result of the psychosis and many psychiatrists would consider that in this case the grounds for termination are considerably strengthened. For example, the wife of a professional man had two children already in their school years. At the age of thirty-eight she developed a schizo-

phrenic illness in which she had the delusion that she should
become pregnant by the devil. As a result, she left the house at
night and consorted with completely unknown men in the local
park. She chose for preference coloured men and soon became
pregnant. It was the pregnancy which led to the discovery of
her delusions which she had managed to conceal previously,
because her husband had been away from home on account
of his work. The problem presented therefore was a patient with
a good home and two normal children who was probably
pregnant by a coloured man as a result of psychotic delusions.
A review of the history suggested there had been some insidious
personality change over a year or two before the onset of the
more acute symptoms. Moreover, since they occurred with
relatively little personality change and apparently little affective
disturbance, it was thought the long-term prognosis was poor.
It was thought that to continue with the pregnancy would
probably reinforce the patient's delusions as she would certainly
live with the knowledge and memory of this episode in her life.
Termination of pregnancy and sterilization were recommended
and the patient also had a course of E.C.T. given sufficiently
frequently to cause a considerable measure of confusion. When
the confusion cleared the patient was left with an amnesia
covering the events leading up to her pregnancy. She therefore
left hospital with the knowledge that she had had a nervous
breakdown and had some permanent loss of memory. She also
knew that during this time she had had an abdominal operation
and was no longer able to have children. Fortunately, her husband was able to give her full support and also arranged his
job to avoid any further periods away from home. Follow-up
after three years showed the patient remained well and con-
tented in a united family.

A history of manic-depressive illness does not carry quite such
a serious import as that of schizophrenia. Neither episodes of
mania or depression lead as a rule to persistent personality
deterioration in the way that schizophrenia may do. Nevertheless, occasionally an episode of mania in a middle-aged woman

may change to a chronic hypomanic state which can be a disaster to the patient and her family. Fortunately this is a rarity. Severe depressions of endogenous type do tend to recur with succeeding childbearing. As noted earlier, the risk tends to be greater with increasing age, therefore should there be one depressive episode following a first child in a young woman, the probability is that she will not have another depression if she becomes pregnant again and one such episode would not, by itself, justify a termination. If, on the other hand, the patient has had two depressive episodes following two pregnancies, then the risks with a third are undoubtedly very considerable. Similarly one depressive episode in an older woman means that with increasing age the risk of further depression following child-bearing is increased. In every case, the total circumstances, in particular the sort of family and the sort of support she can expect from her husband may be crucial. Some account must also be taken of the severity of depression. Where in the past there has clearly been suicidal intent or impulses to harm the baby, these incidents will be taken more seriously than a depression where the patient merely suffers some insom-nia, somatic preoccupation, retardation and general loss of efficiency.

The neuroses present quite a different problem to the psychoses. They are much less easily predicted and tend to occur in the younger patient and by the nature of things, in-cluding the tendency to maturation with age, may well become less frequent as the patient gets older, irrespective of external stress. Many psychiatrists would not regard a neurosis as being an illness of sufficient severity to justify a termination of pregnancy in any case. In the anxiety states for example it is reasonable to assume that the patient will make a good re-covery with or without treatment. On the other hand, some neuroses with phobic symptoms may be precipitated by child-bearing and can persist over many years. A history of such a reaction and eventual recovery might justify consideration of termination of pregnancy. For example a patient with considerable immaturity had developed a severe phobia which prevented her from leaving the house, two months after child-birth. There was a gradual recovery after about two years but the same events were repeated following a second child two years later still. The patient's illness was not reported to her doctor until she was pregnant for the third time and, at this point, her husband insisted that she should get medical advice. An assessment revealed an immature woman who had been over-dependent on her mother. She had married a rather domineering man who had set very high standards. He expected her not only to run the house and bring up the children but to care for his every need. Her phobias developed in a setting of considerable frustration when she found herself unable to manage her baby, the household chores, the shopping and all her husband's demands too. She felt herself to be at fault and regarded herself as a weakling and, therefore, had not con-sidered that medical attention was indicated. The husband wished for a termination of pregnancy on the grounds that his wife's health suffered following childbirth and, though he did not put it quite so frankly, he was considerably inconvenienced when she could not run the household and do the shopping as efficiently as he wished. The patient too asked for a termination of pregnancy but careful discussion with her revealed that this request was made largely to placate her husband, and not from any true depth of desire in herself. Eventually, it was decided not to terminate the pregnancy. The patient was given con-siderable psychotherapy which, unfortunately, had to be restricted once the child was born. A further relapse did occur and phobic symptoms appeared in the third and fourth months following childbirth. At this point a domiciliary visit and further discussion with her husband led to considerable modification of the latter's attitude towards his wife. For the first time, he was able to understand that in her attempts to please him and maintain standards he expected she suffered, and this, in some part, precipitated her symptoms. Once he realized that by supporting, rather than criticizing his wife, she not only felt better but in the long run his own interests were served and a very considerable change in the household took place. On this occasion her phobic symptoms lasted for a much shorter time and it was significant that she matured in the sense that she could accept much more responsibility, could explain herself and her difficulties much more clearly to her husband, and could express some of her resentment towards him. He, in his turn, was able to accept that this show of independence on his wife's part was better for her health and, in the long run, for their mutual happiness.

It has been pointed out that hysteria in the formal sense of the term is a rarity and a patient with severe hysterical symptoms, stemming from considerable inadequacy of personality, is likely to avoid a further pregnancy if, indeed, this played a part in precipitating her symptoms. Histrionic behaviour or emotionally uncontrolled behaviour whether in a patient with a psychopathic personality or from simple immaturity is common and is in no case justification for termination. There is no evidence to suggest that this type of personality defect is worse after childbirth.

Many women become depressed following childbearing but the degree and type of depression does not justify a diagnosis of endogenous depression which implies a psychotic condition. Moreover, many depressions are clearly related in duration and degree to the stress of the patient's life and can be regarded as entirely reactive. In general, since this type of depression may not recur, usually carries a good prognosis and as very often the stress producing it is avoidable, there can be no adequate grounds for recommending a termination of pregnancy. On the other hand, the following case history suggests there may be exceptions. For example, Mrs P. had an unhappy upbringing, her parents quarrelled, the father deserted the family when she was twelve, and her mother was very strict. She had mild episodes of depression in her adolescence, mostly associated with frustrated love affairs. She was eventually courted by a charming psychopath who persuaded her to marry him and promised a satisfactory way of life on the grounds of his regular work and income. Only after marriage did she find he had no regular job and had already spent some time in prison for false pretences. Her married life was punctuated by quarrels with her husband and he deserted her on both occasions when she became pregnant. She was able to rear the two children however and, when they were respectively three and five years of age, her husband was again sent to prison for thieving. He came out of prison a year later, promptly returned home and his wife became pregnant again. At this point, he deserted her once again. She found subsequently that the police were looking for him because of further offences. He was eventually caught and given a further prison sentence. The patient was referred for a psychiatric opinion following a suicide attempt. Examination showed that she was depressed and felt that her present pregnancy made the future hopeless. She could not see how she could maintain her present family with two children now at school, if she were prevented from working because of a pregnancy and new-born child. She suspected from her husband's remarks when he was with her that he intended to desert her and this was eventually confirmed following investigation by the prison doctor. Her husband had been living with another woman at intervals over the previous two or three years. The Health Visitor who knew the patient reported that she was normally an over-conscientious woman, often anxious for her children and tending to fuss over them. In the past she tended to report an excess of minor illnesses and ailments and was over-conscientious with her clinic attendancies. There was no history of previous overt depressive illness other than mood swings in adolescence but her personality structure, together with her present reaction, strongly suggested that a considerable degree of depression with disorganization of her way of life and ability to care for her children was very probable should the pregnancy continue. A termination of pregnancy was recommended and her husband's consent also obtained. Follow-up in this case showed that, in spite of the difficulties of bringing up her children while working, she had maintained her adjustment and there had been no further depression or threat of suicide in the following two years.

The obsessional illnesses can produce very considerable disorganization of the patient's way of life and seriously handicap her and prevent her functioning as a normal wife and mother. Also, as noted earlier, they are frequently of considerable duration and may extend from one pregnancy to the next. If there is a clear history which suggests that previous childbearing precipitated an obsessional illness, this should be considered as a possible justification for termination. Most obsessional patients of course have a very strong sense of what is right and what is wrong, and tend to be somewhat rigid in their observance of what they assume to be expected codes of conduct. In the author's experience, therefore, requests for termination of pregnancy in an obsessional patient are uncommon and tend to occur only in the older patient, particularly if there have been persisting symptoms since a previous child.

It must be emphasized in all cases that not only should the wife and husband's personal opinion be given every possible consideration, but there should be full agreement between the three doctors concerned. Legally, both the patient's consent and that of her husband must be obtained in any case. A possible exception to this is the case of a woman with a florid psychosis as in the one quoted who wished to be pregnant by the devil. In this case, the patient was having treatment under Section 26 of the Mental Health Act and the operation was performed without her written consent but with the consent of her husband and the consultant in charge of the case. Similar action may be necessary in the case of a patient who is a chronic psychotic in a mental hospital who may become pregnant after some years of residence. There may be no next of kin available and the patient may lack insight into the nature of her predicament. In this case, since it is clear her mental state may prevent an adequate assessment of her condition and the risks involved, it is reasonable to state that the patient is unable to make a valid decision because of her mental illness and the decision should be made for her, preferably by the next of kin or by some other responsible person.

Sterilization must be considered seriously in every case where termination of pregnancy is recommended. It should be obvious that where an illness of sufficient severity with the added risk of deterioration in the puerperium is known to exist, that the risk must recur in any succeeding pregnancy, irrespective of when this occurs in a woman's life. It can be argued, particularly in the case of the younger patient, that an illness such as schizophrenia which now carries an uncertain prognosis may, as a result of changes in treatment, carry a very good prognosis in the foreseeable future. Nevertheless, in most cases where termination is recommended, a sterilization is also necessary. This may also be true in general medicine but is particularly the case in psychiatry. Very often the mental illness which makes the patient liable to deterioration after childbearing may also make her less able to use common methods of birth-control. Moreover, most methods of birth-control have a small failure rate, even in the intelligent and co-operative patient. Most women and their doctors are even more averse to a termination than to a sterilization and many women will accept a sterilization who would not accept a termination, should this be recommended at a later stage. Where the patient already has, say, two children, and a termination is recommended, sterilization should be the rule. On the other hand, if the patient has no children or one child, and is still young, there may be some uncertainty and each case must be decided on its merits. For example, a young woman with a hebephrenic type of schizophrenia who already has one child would be well advised to have a sterilization so that the risk of further deterioration and personality loss will be avoided for ever. Moreover, with this type of illness she is likely to find child-rearing a strain and one child may be the maximum that her capabilities will allow. On the other hand, a patient with a history of depression, even if severe, following one child, may become pregnant under conditions of considerable stress. For example, her husband may be in the services and have an overseas posting This could lead to the possibility of termination being considered if she is likely to have the child during his absence. On the other hand, since it might be possible for them to plan a child when he has a home posting again or under conditions when they are united and she will get some supervision from a reliable relative during the puerperium, it is conceivable that a termination could be indicated, but no sterilization performed.

Some patients with a neurosis have specific fears of childbearing. They may indeed have one or two children or none at all but in some of these patients severe anxiety states persist with exacerbation in each pre-menstrual phase as the patient becomes increasingly preoccupied with the fear that she may be pregnant. There will be some temporary relief with each period and the cycle then recurs. Certainly psychotherapy and other methods of treatment should be attempted but some of these patients have such persistent fears and so few personality resources that a sterilization may be justified as the only step likely to lead to permanent relief of this particular fear.

Index